ADVANCE PRAISE FOR *A CLINICIAN'S GUIDE TO DISCLOSURES OF SEXUAL ASSAULT*

"This book is an essential resource for clinicians working with sexual assault survivors. Based on the latest research, the authors provide an accessible overview of what is known about sexual assault disclosure and social reactions and how it can be used in clinical treatment with survivors of differing backgrounds and experiences."

—**Sarah E. Ullman**, PhD,
Professor of Criminology & Psychology,
University of Illinois at Chicago

"*A Clinician's Guide to Disclosures of Sexual Assault* by Amie R. Newins and Laura C. Wilson fills a niche that has been needed. How to elicit and handle disclosures of sexual assault appropriately and sensitively with a wide variety of population groups is an important resource for all service providers to read. This book is recommended to a wide range of professions and may prevent further damage and could elicit the beginning of the healing process among those who have been sexually assaulted."

—**Patricia A. Resick**, PhD, ABPP,
Professor of Psychiatry and Behavioral Sciences,
Duke Health

T0323423

ABCT Clinical Practice Series

Series Editor

Susan W. White, Ph.D., ABPP, Professor and Doddridge Saxon Chair in Clinical Psychology, University of Alabama

Associate Editors

Lara J. Farrell, Ph.D., Associate Professor, School of Applied Psychology, Griffith University & Menzies Health Institute of Queensland, Australia

Matthew A. Jarrett, Ph.D., Associate Professor, Department of Psychology, University of Alabama

Jordana Muroff, Ph.D., LICSW, Associate Professor, Clinical Practice, Boston University School of Social Work

Marisol Perez, Ph.D., Associate Professor & Associate Chair, Department of Psychology, Arizona State University

Titles in the Series

A Clinician's Guide to Disclosures of Sexual Assault

AMIE R. NEWINS

AND

LAURA C. WILSON

OXFORD
UNIVERSITY PRESS

OXFORD
UNIVERSITY PRESS

Oxford University Press is a department of the University of Oxford. It furthers
the University's objective of excellence in research, scholarship, and education
by publishing worldwide. Oxford is a registered trade mark of Oxford University
Press in the UK and certain other countries.

Published in the United States of America by Oxford University Press
198 Madison Avenue, New York, NY 10016, United States of America.

© Oxford University Press 2021

Library of Congress Cataloging-in-Publication Data
Names: Newins, Amie R., author | Wilson, Laura C., author.
Title: A clinician's guide to disclosures of sexual assault / Amie R. Newins, Laura C. Wilson.
Description: New York, NY : Oxford University Press, [2021] |
Series: ABCT clinical practice series | Includes bibliographical references and index.
Identifiers: LCCN 2021012737 (print) | LCCN 2021012738 (ebook) |
ISBN 9780197523643 (paperback) | ISBN 9780197523667 (epub) | ISBN 9780197523674
Subjects: LCSH: Rape victims—United States. | Rape victims—
Services for—United States. | Sexual abuse victims—United States. |
Sexual abuse victims—Services for—United States.
Classification: LCC HV6561 .N49 2021 (print) | LCC HV6561 (ebook) |
DDC 362.88392/630973—dc23
LC record available at https://lccn.loc.gov/2021012737
LC ebook record available at https://lccn.loc.gov/2021012738

DOI: 10.1093/med-psych/9780197523643.001.0001

9 8 7 6 5 4 3 2 1

Printed by Marquis, Canada

CONTENTS

FOREWORD

Mental health clinicians desperately want to help their clients, and recognize the importance of implementing evidence-based treatments toward achieving this goal. In the past several years, the field of mental health care has seen tremendous advances in our understanding of pathology and its underlying mechanisms, as well as proliferation and refinement of scientifically informed treatment approaches. Coinciding with these advances is a heightened focus on accountability in clinical practice. Clinicians are expected to apply evidence-based approaches, and to do so effectively, efficiently, and in a patient-centered, individualized way. This is no small order. For a multitude of reasons, including but not limited to client diversity, complex psychopathology (e.g., comorbidity), and barriers to care that are not under the clinician's control (e.g., adverse life circumstances that limit the client's ability to participate), delivery of evidence-based approaches can be challenging.

This series, which represents a collaborative effort between the Association for Behavioral and Cognitive Therapies (ABCT) and the Oxford University Press, is intended to serve as an easy-to-use, highly practical collection of resources for clinicians and trainees. The *ABCT Clinical Practice Series* is designed to help clinicians effectively master and implement evidence-based treatment approaches. In practical terms, the series represents the "brass tacks" of implementation, including basic how-to guidance and advice on troubleshooting common issues in clinical practice and application. As such, the series is best viewed as a complement to other series on evidence-based protocols such as the *Treatments That Work*™ series and the *Programs That Work*™ series. These represent seminal bridges between research and practice, and have been instrumental in the dissemination of empirically supported intervention protocols and programs. The *ABCT Clinical Practice Series*, rather than focusing on specific diagnoses and their treatment, targets the practical application of therapeutic and assessment approaches. In other words, the emphasis is on the *how-to* aspects of mental health delivery.

It is my hope that clinicians and trainees find these books useful in refining their clinical skills, as enhanced comfort as well as competence in delivery of evidence-based approaches should ultimately lead to improved client outcomes. Given the emphasis on application in this series, there is relatively less emphasis on review of the underlying research base. Readers who wish to delve more deeply into the theoretical or empirical basis supporting specific approaches are encouraged to go to the original source publications cited in each chapter. When relevant, suggestions for further reading are provided.

Given the unfortunately high prevalence of sexual assault across countries and cultures, all mental health care providers. including those who do not "specialize" in trauma, must be prepared to sensitively address client disclosures. In this timely volume, *A Clinician's Guide to Disclosures of Sexual Assault*, Dr. Amie R. Newins and Dr. Laura C. Wilson provide clinicians and trainees with information to help be prepared for this eventuality. They synthesize the extant research on predictors and consequences of disclosure, assault risk, and survivorship, and provide guidance on how to therapeutically address disclosures of sexual assault based on their many years of clinical and research experience in this area.

While there are several excellent books focused on the treatment of PTSD and sexual assault specifically, this is the first book that was developed explicitly to provide clinicians with specific guidance on how to handle disclosures of sexual assault. As such, this is sure to be a valuable book for graduate clinical courses, including practicum training.

Susan W. White, PhD, ABPP
Series Editor

Scope of the Issue

Prevalence of Sexual Assault, Psychosocial Consequences, and Survivor Disclosure

Sexual assault survivors[1] face a precarious dilemma regarding whether or not to disclose their experience. Many survivors, once they disclose their victimization to others, are met with support and validation. These survivors report better outcomes. Unfortunately, others are not believed or are blamed for the incident(s). These negative reactions can have devastating consequences on their long-term recovery. The uncertainty of how others will respond to them leaves many sexual assault survivors hesitant to report their victimization to the authorities, tell friends or family, or seek mental or physical health services. Simply put, the people who surround sexual assault survivors have an instrumental role in facilitating their recovery.

With this in mind, the aim of this book is to provide guidance on how to interact with survivors of sexual assault. The content is applicable to professionals in a range of settings including, but not limited to, mental health, physical health, education, law, victim services, and the military. As a consequence of numerous events, such as the MeToo movement and the "Dear Colleague letter" issued by the U.S. Department of Education, the rate of disclosure among survivors has been increasing. It is paramount that professionals in all relevant fields be prepared to offer appropriate emotional and practical support to sexual assault survivors. Professionals who are comfortable with and skilled in providing services competently to sexual assault survivors are an important part of ensuring they receive the validation and empowerment they deserve.

From the outset, we would like to make the reader aware that prior studies conducted on sexual assault have, to this point, disproportionately focused on survivors who are White, female, and currently in college. Additionally, the

---

1. Throughout this book, we use the term "victim" when writing about the time period during the crime and the term "survivor" when referencing any time period after the crime. See Chapter 2 for a more thorough discussion of these terms and the importance of language.

majority of the literature fails to take into account other potentially relevant aspects of identity, which ultimately results in bias in the literature, such as heteronormativity and cisnormativity. Given that sexual assault can impact people far beyond these particular demographic characteristics, there is certainly more work to do to better understand the range of experiences among survivors, and this should be of great priority for scholars who engage in this type of work. Furthermore, we encourage readers to keep this limitation of the literature in mind when reading this book because the themes and trends identified do not necessarily reflect all survivors. We further discuss issues that are relevant to working with particular populations of survivors in Chapter 9.

DEFINITION OF SEXUAL ASSAULT

In this book, we define sexual assault as sexual contact or penetration without the explicit consent of the victim. Therefore, we use sexual assault as an umbrella term that encompasses a wide range of sexual violence incidents, such as unwanted fondling, oral sex, and vaginal and anal penetration. We have provided this definition to clarify the scope of the book, but we would also like to offer a disclaimer about definitions within the context of working with sexual assault survivors. While definitions that differentiate between types of sexual violence are useful in the domains of research and law, when you are working face to face with clients in other settings (e.g., clinical and educational settings), their utility is attenuated and may even be counterproductive. For example, as we will discuss in Chapter 2, rape survivors rarely use the word "rape" to describe what happened to them (Wilson & Miller, 2016). Therefore, clients may deny experiencing sexual assault if professionals are restricted in how they talk about victimization or they may be resistant if professionals push certain words on them. The use of strict definitions also perpetuates the "real rape" stereotype or the idea that in order for sexual victimization to be considered "real," it has to satisfy certain criteria (Temkin & Krahe, 2008). In fact, no two experiences of sexual assault are the same, and professionals are advised to be flexible and open-minded in their interactions with clients in terms of terminology and definitions (Worell & Remer, 1992). We will further discuss issues related to language in Chapter 2.

PREVALENCE OF SEXUAL ASSAULT

National data indicate that approximately one in three women and one in six men in the United States experience contact sexual violence during their lifetime (Smith et al., 2017). However, because the measures typically used (e.g., climate surveys on college campuses) do not capture incidents that are often perceived as "milder" (e.g., someone rubbing against you without your permission), it is possible that prevalence rates of sexual violence are even higher (Papp & McClelland, 2020). Although the exact prevalence of sexual violence varies across countries, the frequency worldwide has led to sexual violence being deemed a serious public health issue (Krug et al., 2002). Thus, there are robust data that suggest sexual violence is a pervasive problem, which highlights the importance of professionals across fields being ready to talk to survivors about sexual assault in an affirming and supportive way.

Research has also revealed that some individuals may be at disproportionately heightened risk of sexual assault. For example, in the United States, American Indian/Alaska Native and multiracial women report higher rates of contact sexual violence (45.6% and 49.5%, respectively) compared to women of other races and ethnicities (22.9% to 38.9%; Smith et al., 2017). Men in the United States followed a similar pattern, with American Indian/Alaska Native and multiracial men reporting higher rates of contact sexual violence (23.1% and 31.9%, respectively) compared to men of other races and ethnicities (9.4% to 19.4%; Smith et al., 2017). Individuals who identify as gay, lesbian, and bisexual, as well as other members of the sexual minority community, have also been found to be at heightened risk of sexual assault across their lifespan compared to individuals who identify as heterosexual (Rothman et al., 2011), with the highest rates among women who identify as bisexual (Ford & Soto-Marquez, 2016). Gender identity has also been linked to level of risk. For example, a study showed that individuals who identify as transgender (20.9%) had significantly greater risk of sexual violence in the past year compared to cisgender women (8.6%) and cisgender men (3.6%; Coulter et al., 2017). The rate of victimization was even higher among Black individuals who identified as transgender (55.6%; Coulter et al., 2017). These findings highlight the need for an intersectional framework and for professionals to have an adequate level of cultural competence to understand how multiple aspects of identity can compound one's risk for sexual violence.

It is important to note that group differences in rates of sexual violence, such as those reviewed here, reflect differences in risk mechanisms and do not indicate that aspects of identity, such as race or sexual orientation, are inherent or direct causes of increased risk for sexual assault. For example, Thompson et al. (2012) found that racial and ethnic differences in sexual assault risk could be partially explained by observed differences in substance use. When group differences are demonstrated, professionals should consider the mechanisms driving those trends because that information could potentially inform intervention. Furthermore, professionals need to be careful to monitor any potential stereotypes they hold about working with certain groups of individuals or in certain settings because those beliefs could impact their ability to engage in a respectful, unbiased professional relationship with clients. We will review this topic more in Chapters 9 and 10.

There are also several specific settings that should be of particular focus when discussing sexual violence, including the military, higher education, and correctional facilities. In recent years, the military has increasingly become concerned about the rates of sexual violence and misconduct among service members and has taken actions to improve prevention measures, assessment of sexual assault, investigation procedures, and support of survivors. A meta-analysis demonstrated that 15.7% of military personnel and veterans (38.4% of women, 3.9% of men) experience military sexual trauma during their service, which includes both sexual assault and harassment (Wilson, 2018). Furthermore, data suggest that reports of sexual assault and harassment in the military have been increasing in recent years. Specifically, from 2018 to 2019 there was a 3% increase in reports of sexual assault and a 10% increase in reports of sexual harassment (Department of Defense, 2020). These data do not necessarily reflect an increase in the base rate of military sexual trauma; rather, they may indicate that rates of disclosures are increasing. What is particularly noteworthy is that confidential disclosures increased 17% during that time period (Department of Defense, 2020). This type of reporting indicates that the survivor does not want to initiate an official investigation at that time, which could mean that they are concerned about how they would be treated (e.g., retaliation) or how the case would be handled (e.g., case details would be made public). Furthermore, research conducted within the Veterans Health Administration has shown that both male and female veterans are hesitant to seek services because of apprehension about being able to trust their provider and concerns that they will be judged (Monteith et al., 2020). Overall, the evidence is clear that the rate of disclosures of military sexual trauma is on the rise and more work is needed to ensure survivors feel safe and supported during the reporting process and when seeking services.

Similar to the military, there has been increased scrutiny of the rates of sexual violence on college and university campuses in the United States over the past decade. This concern was evident in the "Dear Colleague letter" issued by the U.S. Department of Education in April 2011, which called attention to the high rates of sexual violence among college students and clarified expectations of how schools should handle the assessment, investigation, and documentation of incidents (Ali, 2011). A large national survey of colleges and universities found that 13% of students had experienced nonconsensual sexual contact, with women, individuals who identify as transgender and non-binary, and undergraduate students reporting higher rates than men, cisgender individuals, and graduate students, respectively (Cantor et al., 2019). Furthermore, among schools that participated in both the 2015 and 2019 surveys, the rate of sexual violence had increased over those years. As discussed in reference to the military, this increase could reflect an actual increase in occurrence. However, it could also reflect other changes, such as increased awareness, which could have led more survivors to feel comfortable participating in this type of a survey. Also similar to the data reported by the military, students have concerns about how reports and investigations of sexual assault will be handled. Although 66% of students said they thought school officials would take reports of sexual assault seriously, the percentage dropped to 45% among students who had actually experienced nonconsensual sexual contact (Cantor et al., 2019). It is apparent that all higher education employees (e.g., faculty, campus police, residence life staff) need to be increasingly prepared to receive disclosures of sexual violence and school officials need to improve training and policies to make this process as survivor-centered and affirming as possible. Sexual violence is an issue that needs a comprehensive approach involving all entities on campuses, and therefore sexual violence training and resources should not be restricted to campus counseling centers and Title IX offices.

Compared to the military and college campuses, underreporting of sexual violence may be an even bigger issue in correctional facilities. For example, it has been estimated that only about 8% of prisoners who experience sexual victimization during their incarceration report the incident to prison officials (Beck et al., 2010; Guerino & Beck, 2011). Many factors contribute to whether or not prisoners report their victimization, including systemic inequalities and power imbalances. However, other factors need to be considered. For example, most assaults in prison do not involve physical injury, which may lead prisoners to think that prison officials will take the report less seriously (Beck et al., 2013; Owen et al., 2008). Furthermore, prisoners may receive goods or protection from their perpetrator(s) and therefore may be less likely to report the incident(s) out of fear that they will no longer receive those advantages (Owen et al., 2008). Prisoners may also witness others' reports of sexual violence go unsubstantiated and therefore think it is futile to report their own victimization. Because of underreporting, it is extremely challenging to obtain an accurate estimate of how common sexual violence is in prisons and jails. The U.S. Department of Justice reported that the number of allegations of sexual victimization in prisons and jails nearly tripled from 2011 to 2015 (8,768 were reported in 2011 compared to 24,661 in 2015; Rantala, 2018). Regardless of the exact prevalence of sexual violence in correctional facilities, it is well understood that many of the issues sexual violence survivors face in the community are exacerbated when the violence occurs behind bars. To be effective disclosure recipients, employees in these facilities need to be well versed in the unique challenges that incarcerated survivors face.

Overall, the data suggest that, regardless of setting, disclosures of sexual assault are increasing. There is also evidence that survivors, again regardless of setting, have concerns about how official reports of sexual assault will be handled, which impacts the likelihood that they will disclose what happened to formal sources of support. Given that existing research shows huge discrepancies between official reports of sexual victimization and prevalence rates obtained through confidential surveys (Beck et al., 2010; Guerino & Beck, 2011), it is vital that professionals in all settings conduct anonymous or confidential surveys to get a sense of the level of underreporting that is occurring and to identify the obstacles from the perspective of the survivors. More information about special considerations for working with particular populations of sexual assault survivors will be provided in Chapter 9.

PSYCHOSOCIAL OUTCOMES OF SEXUAL ASSAULT

There is an extensive literature base demonstrating that many sexual assault survivors experience a range of difficulties. For the purposes of this book, we will simply review some of the more relevant findings. In terms of posttraumatic stress disorder (PTSD), survivors of rape and other forms of sexual assault have a higher risk of developing PTSD compared to all other types of trauma (e.g., war-related trauma, accidents, physical violence; Kessler et al., 2017). Although PTSD is the most commonly discussed psychological disorder in relation to sexual assault, the mental health consequences of sexual assault also include other forms of psychopathology, such as depression, anxiety, and substance misuse (Dworkin et al., 2017; Mechanic, 2004). Furthermore, to truly capture the outcomes of survivors, professionals need to consider a range of other difficulties, including but not limited to poor academic performance, reduced productivity at work, interpersonal difficulties, physical health conditions, and increased risk of future sexual victimization (i.e., revictimization; Jordan et al., 2014; Mechanic, 2004; Smith & Breiding, 2011; Walker et al., 2019). Additionally, many survivors do not present for services until several years after their victimization experience (Thompson, 2000). As a result, it is important for mental health providers to assess each survivor's mental health symptoms and provide services appropriate for those difficulties. Furthermore, some survivors who need trauma-focused treatment may not be ready to engage in that treatment, and providers should be prepared to offer or refer to treatment to help prepare survivors for trauma-focused treatment. More information related to psychotherapy is provided in Chapter 5.

It is also important to keep in mind that a comprehensive assessment is necessary to determine all factors that are contributing to a survivor's level of functioning. For example, many male survivors report that their victimization undermines their masculinity (Weiss, 2010), child sexual abuse may exacerbate the effects of later victimization (Briere et al., 2020), many sexual and gender minority survivors report an extensive history of discrimination and prejudice (e.g., heterosexism, transphobia; Meyer, 2003), and racial minority survivors may evidence poorer mental health and physical health outcomes because of systemic inequalities (Garcia & Rivera, 2014). More issues related to assessment will be discussed in Chapter 4, and special considerations for working with particular populations will be discussed in Chapter 9.

It is also important to know that a growing literature base has demonstrated that some survivors experience posttraumatic growth, which is positive psychological change that stems from enduring the trauma (e.g., feeling closer to others, feeling a greater sense of purpose; Frazier & Berman, 2008). Being aware of the potential for posttraumatic growth can have a positive impact on both providers and survivors because it fosters hope and resiliency (Thompson, 2000). Finally, providers need to be mindful that posttraumatic recovery among survivors is rarely, if ever, linear. In fact, symptoms tend to ebb and flow, and survivors may simultaneously experience indicators of posttraumatic growth (e.g., feeling a greater sense of purpose) and psychopathology (e.g., sleep difficulties, depressed mood; Kelly et al., 1996). It is important to validate this process for survivors and to ensure they have realistic expectations about outcomes. For example, many survivors present to therapy with the hope of being "cured" of their depression or PTSD. This hope could be problematic because survivors may become frustrated by their inability to achieve that goal, which can exacerbate their difficulties. Instead, providers should work with clients to develop realistic treatment goals and provide psychoeducation on the psychosocial impact of sexual assault, including recognition of the possibility of posttraumatic growth. Overall, to truly offer survivor-centered support and services, professionals need to recognize that outcomes follow unique trajectories and thorough, unbiased assessment is needed to adequately capture the survivor's presenting problem(s) and their person-specific contributing factors.

INFORMAL AND FORMAL DISCLOSURES

For the purposes of this book, we will define a disclosure as any time a sexual assault survivor reveals to either an informal (e.g., family member, friend) or formal (e.g., police, therapist) source that they have been victimized. Survivors may disclose for a wide variety of reasons, including to obtain tangible assistance (e.g., seek medical services) or emotional support (e.g., validation). Numerous factors have contributed to a recent increase in disclosures, with the MeToo movement being one of the most visible (Alaggia & Wang, 2020; Bogen et al., 2019). The MeToo movement, which was founded by activist Tarana Burke in 2006 and became a trending hashtag (#MeToo) in 2017, ignited a worldwide conversation about the prevalence and consequences of sexual violence. This social media movement increased awareness about sexual violence among the general population and helped many survivors find their voice in sharing their own experiences and make meaning of what happened to them (Alaggia & Wang, 2020). The MeToo movement certainly should be celebrated as a step in the right direction in terms of amplifying the stories of survivors and increasing public awareness about sexual violence. However, another aspect of the movement needs to be examined: Numerous studies have suggested that sexual assault survivors have turned to online platforms because they have failed to find support through other avenues (Moors & Webber, 2012). This issue is especially troublesome because survivors do in fact report receiving mixed reactions from professionals, particularly in the legal setting (Alaggia & Wang, 2020). While online activity, such as posting and receiving responses via social media, is an emerging and potentially positive avenue through which survivors can receive support (Alaggia & Wang, 2020), it is unacceptable if survivors view this activity as the only means through which they can receive affirmation. It is on professionals to earn the trust and confidence of sexual assault survivors.

Generally speaking, most survivors disclose their sexual assault to at least one informal source of support, typically within the first few weeks following the incident (Orchowski & Gidycz, 2012; Sylaska & Edwards, 2014). Disclosures to formal sources of support, such as therapists and police officers, are less common and are perceived by survivors as less helpful and more harmful than disclosures to informal sources (Filipas & Ullman, 2001; Ullman & Filipas, 2001). Furthermore, it is not just sexual assault survivors who view reactions from formal sources as potentially problematic. When randomly surveyed, most licensed mental health professionals reported that they believe that other mental health professionals are engaging in harmful practices with sexual assault survivors (Campbell & Raja,

1999). The fear of these negative reactions contributes to survivors' resistance to disclose their victimization, which can serve as an obstacle to seeking needed services or reporting the crime (Ullman & Filipas, 2001). For example, only 17% of women who experience sexual assault report it to the police (Sloan et al., 1997), only 7% seek help from mental health providers (Ullman, 1996), and between 5% and 10% seek services from rape crisis centers (Golding et al., 1989). These low rates of crime reporting and service seeking are concerning and addressing them should be of the highest priority among professionals in these fields.

CONCLUSION

As a society, we have recently made great gains in our conversation about sexual assault. Survivors are increasingly coming forward and sharing their stories. The general population is more educated about the rate at which sexual violence occurs, as well as about the devastating and far-reaching consequences this form of violence can have on people. The field is more informed on the range of psychosocial outcomes that survivors can experience, and scholars better appreciate the unique trajectories of recovery displayed by survivors. We are more informed and more aware, as a whole. Unfortunately, survivors still experience obstacles to reporting victimization and seeking competent services. In the remaining chapters of this book, we will highlight some of the common issues that emerge when working with sexual assault survivors and we will offer best practices with the goal of making services more survivor-centered.

REFERENCES

Alaggia, R., & Wang, S. (2020). "I never told anyone until the #metoo movement": What can we learn from sexual abuse and sexual assault disclosures made through social media? *Child Abuse & Neglect, 103*, Article 104312. https://doi.org/10.1016/j.chiabu.2019.104312

Ali, R. (2011). *Dear colleague letter.* U.S. Department of Education, Office for Civil Rights. https://www2.ed.gov/about/offices/list/ocr/letters/colleague-201104.pdf

Beck, A., Berzofsky, M., Caspar, R., & Krebs, C. (2013). *Sexual victimization in prisons and jails reported by inmates, 2011–12.* U.S. Department of Justice, Bureau of Justice Statistics. https://www.bjs.gov/content/pub/pdf/svpjri1112.pdf

Beck, A. J., Harrison, P. M., Berzofsky, M., Caspar, R., & Krebs, C. (2010). *Sexual victimization in prisons and jails reported by inmates, 2008–09.* U.S. Department of Justice, Bureau of Justice Statistics. https://www.bjs.gov/content/pub/pdf/svpjri0809.pdf

Bogen, K. W., Bleiweiss, K. K., Leach, N. R., & Orchowski, L. M. (2019). #MeToo: Disclosure and response to sexual victimization on Twitter. *Journal of Interpersonal Violence.* Advance online publication. https://doi.org/10.1177/0886260519851211

Briere, J., Runtz, M., Rassart, C. A., Rodd, K., & Godbout, N. (2020). Sexual assault trauma: Does prior childhood maltreatment increase the risk and exacerbate the outcome? *Child Abuse & Neglect, 103,* Article 104421. https://doi.org/10.1016/j.chiabu.2020.104421

Campbell, R., & Raja, S. (1999). Secondary victimization of rape victims: Insights from mental health professionals who treat survivors of violence. *Violence and Victims, 14*(3), 261–275. https://doi.org/10.1891/0886-6708.14.3.261

Cantor, D., Fisher, B., Chibnall, S., Harps, S., Townsend, R., Thomas, G., Lee, H., Kranz, V., Herbison, R., & Madden, K. (2019). *Report on the AAU campus climate survey on sexual assault and misconduct.* https://www.aau.edu/sites/default/files/AAU-Files/Key-Issues/Campus-Safety/Revised%20Aggregate%20report%20%20and%20appendices%201-7_(01-16-2020_FINAL).pdf

Coulter, R. W. S., Mair, C., Miller, E., Blosnich, J. R., Matthews, D. D., & McCauley, H. L. (2017). Prevalence of past-year sexual assault victimization among undergraduate students: Exploring differences by and intersections of gender identity, sexual identity, and race/ethnicity. *Prevention Science, 18*(6), 726–736. https://doi.org/10.1007/s11121-017-0762-8

Department of Defense. (2020). *Department of Defense annual report on sexual assault in the military: Fiscal year 2019.* https://media.defense.gov/2020/Apr/30/2002291660/-1/-1/1/1_department_of_defense_fiscal_year_2019_annual_report_on_sexual_assault_in_the_military.PDF

Dworkin, E. R., Menon, S. V., Bystrynski, J., & Allen, N. E. (2017). Sexual assault victimization and psychopathology: A review and meta-analysis. *Clinical Psychology Review, 56,* 65–81. https://doi.org/10.1016/j.cpr.2017.06.002

Filipas, H. H., & Ullman, S. E. (2001). Social reactions to sexual assault victims from various support sources. *Violence and Victims, 16*(6), 673–692.

Ford, J., & Soto-Marquez, J. (2016). Sexual assault victimization among straight, gay/lesbian, and bisexual college students. *Violence & Gender, 3*(2), 107–115. https://doi.org/10.1089/vio.2015.0030

Frazier, P. A., & Berman, M. I. (2008). Posttraumatic growth following sexual assault. In S. Joseph & P. A. Linley (Eds.), *Trauma, recovery, and growth: Positive psychological perspectives on posttraumatic stress* (pp.161–184). Wiley & Sons.

Garcia, G., & Rivera, M. (2014). Is race a factor in disparate health problems associated with violence against women? *Journal of Health Disparities Research and Practice, 7*(2), 10–23. https://digitalscholarship.unlv.edu/cgi/viewcontent.cgi?article=1221&context=jhdrp

Golding, J. M., Siegel, J. M., Sorenson, S. B., Burnam, M. A., & Stein, J. A. (1989). Social support sources following sexual assault. *Journal of Community Psychology, 17*(1), 92–107. https://doi.org/10.1002/1520-6629(198901)17:1<92::AID-JCOP2290170110>3.0.CO;2-E

Guerino, P., & Beck, A. J. (2011). *Sexual victimization reported by adult correctional authorities, 2007–2008.* U.S. Department of Justice, Office of Justice Programs, Bureau of Justice Statistics. https://www.bjs.gov/content/pub/pdf/svraca0911.pdf

Jordan, C. E., Combs, J. L., & Smith, G. T. (2014). An exploration of sexual victimization and academic performance among college women. *Trauma, Violence, & Abuse, 15*(3), 191–200. https://doi.org/10.1177/1524838014520637

Kelly, L., Burton, S., & Regan, L. (1996). Beyond victim or survivor: Sexual violence, identity and feminist theory and practice. In L. Adkins & V. Merchant (Eds.), *Sexualizing the social: Power and the organization of sexuality* (pp. 77–101). St. Martin's Press.

Kessler, R. C., Aguilar-Gaxiola, S., Alonso, J., Benjet, C., Bromet, E. J., Cardoso, G., Degenhardt, L., de Girolamo, G., Dinolova, R. V., Ferry, F., Florescu, S., Gureje, O., Haro, J. M., Huang, Y., Karam, E. G., Kawakami, N., Lee, S., Lepine, J.-P., Levinson, D., . . . WHO World Mental Health Survey Collaborators. (2017). Trauma and PTSD in the WHO world mental health surveys. *European Journal of Psychotraumatology*, 8(Suppl 5), 1353383. https://doi.org/10.1080/20008198.2017.1353383

Krug, E. G., Dahlberg, L. L., Mercy, J. A., Zwi, A. B., & Lozano, R. (2002). *World report on violence and health*. World Health Organization. https://www.who.int/violence_injury_prevention/violence/world_report/en/summary_en.pdf

Mechanic, M. (2004). Beyond PTSD: Mental health consequences of violence against women: A response to Briere and Jordan. *Journal of Interpersonal Violence*, 19(11), 1283–1289. https://doi.org/10.1177/0886260504270690

Meyer, I. H. (2003). Prejudice, social stress, and mental health in lesbian, gay, and bisexual populations: Conceptual issues and research evidence. *Psychological Bulletin*, 129(5), 674–697. https://doi.org/10.1037/0033-2909.129.5.674

Monteith, L. L., Bahraini, N. H., Gerber, H. R., Holliman, B. D., Schneider, A. L., Holliday, R., & Matarazzo, B. B. (2020). Military sexual trauma survivors' perceptions of veterans health administration care: A qualitative examination. *Psychological Services*, 17(2), 178–186. https://doi.org/10.1037/ser0000290

Moors, R., & Webber, R. (2012). The dance of disclosure: On-line disclosure of sexual assault. *Qualitative Social Work*, 12(6), 799–815. https://doi.org/10.1177/1473325012464383

Orchowski, L. M., & Gidycz, C. A. (2012). To whom do college women confide following sexual assault? A prospective study of predictors of sexual assault disclosure and social reactions. *Violence Against Women*, 18(3), 264–288. https://doi.org/10.1177/1077801212442917

Owen, B. A., Wells, J., Pollock, J., Muscat, B., & Torres, S. (2008). *Gendered violence and safety: A contextual approach to improving security in women's facilities*. California State University Press. https://www.ncjrs.gov/pdffiles1/nij/grants/225338.pdf

Papp, L. J., & McClelland, S. I. (2020). Too common to count? "Mild" sexual assault and aggression among U.S. college women. *Journal of Sex Research*. Advance online publication. https://doi.org/10.1080/00224499.2020.1778620

Rantala, R. R. (2018). *Sexual victimization reported by adult correctional authorities, 2012-2015*. U.S. Department of Justice, Bureau of Justice Statistics. https://www.bjs.gov/index.cfm?ty=pbdetail&iid=6326

Rothman, E. F., Exner, D., & Baughman, A. (2011). The prevalence of sexual assault against people who identify as gay, lesbian or bisexual in the United States: A systematic review. *Trauma, Violence, & Abuse*, 12(2), 55–66. https://doi.org/10.1177/1524838010390707.

Sloan, J. J., Fisher, B. S., & Cullen, F. T. (1997). Assessing the student right-to-know and Campus Security Act of 1990: An analysis of the victim reporting practices of college and university students. *Crime and Delinquency*, 43(2), 148–168. https://doi.org/10.1177/0011128797043002002

Smith, S. G., & Breiding, M. J. (2011). Chronic disease and health behaviours linked to experiences of non-consensual sex among women and men. *Public Health*, 125(9), 653–659. https://doi.org/10.1016/j.puhe.2011.06.006

Smith, S. G., Chen, J., Basile, K. C., Gilbert, L. K., Merrick, M. T., Patel, N., Walling, M., & Jain, A. (2017). *The National Intimate Partner and Sexual Violence Survey (NISVS): 2010–2012 State Report*. Centers for Disease Control and Prevention, National Center for Injury Prevention and Control. https://www.cdc.gov/violenceprevention/pdf/nisvs-statereportbook.pdf

Sylaska, K. M., & Edwards, K. M. (2014). Disclosure of intimate partner violence to informal social support network members: A review of the literature. *Trauma, Violence, & Abuse, 15*(1), 3–21. https://doi.org/10.1177/1524838013496335

Temkin, J., & Krahe, B. (2008). *Sexual assault and the justice gap: A question of attitude*. Hart Publishing.

Thompson, M. (2000). Life after rape: A chance to speak? *Sexual and Relationship Therapy, 15*(4), 325–343. https://doi.org/10.1080/713697439

Thompson, N. J., McGee, R. E., & Mays, D. (2012). Race, ethnicity, substance use, and unwanted sexual intercourse among adolescent females in the United States. *Western Journal of Emergency Medicine, 13*(3), 283–288. https://doi.org/10.5811/westjem.2012.3.11774

Ullman, S. E. (1996). Social reactions, coping strategies, and self-blame attributions in adjustment to sexual assault. *Psychology of Women Quarterly, 20*(4), 505–526. https://doi.org/10.1111/j.1471-6402.1996.tb00319.x

Ullman, S. E., & Filipas, H. H. (2001). Correlates of formal and informal support seeking in sexual assault victims. *Journal of Interpersonal Violence, 16*(10), 1028–1047. https://doi.org/10.1177%2F088626001016010004

Walker, H. E., Freud, J. S., Ellis, R. A., Fraine, S. M., & Wilson, L. C. (2019). The prevalence of sexual revictimization: A meta-analytic review. *Trauma, Violence, & Abuse, 20*(1), 67–80. https://doi.org/10.1177/1524838017692364

Weiss, K. G. (2010). Male sexual victimization: Examining men's experiences of rape and sexual assault. *Men and Masculinities, 12*(3), 275–298. https://doi.org/10.1177/1097184X08322632

Wilson, L. C. (2018). The prevalence of military sexual trauma: A meta-analysis. *Trauma, Violence, & Abuse, 19*(5), 584–597. https://doi.org/10.1177/1524838016683459

Wilson, L. C., & Miller, K. E. (2016). Meta-analysis of the prevalence of unacknowledged rape. *Trauma, Violence, & Abuse, 17*(2), 149–159. https://doi.org/10.1177/1524838015576391

Worell, J., & Remer, P. (1992). *Feminist perspective in therapy: An empowerment model for women*. John Wiley & Sons.

2

Labels and Language Related to Sexual Assault

Professionals need to critically consider the language they use when working with sexual assault survivors. For example, the words professionals choose can shape how others perceive an incident, reveal their own assumptions and biases to others, privilege some survivors over others, and communicate that some forms of victimization should be considered more serious than others. Language is a powerful tool that can convey the professional is an empathic helper; such language will encourage survivors to seek services and disclose their victimization. Conversely, if problematic (e.g., labeling, dismissive) language is used, professionals may inadvertently alienate survivors or exacerbate the difficulties they face (e.g., self-blame, embarrassment). Given that survivors overestimate the extent to which others believe rape myths (Paul et al., 2009), intentional work focused on the language that professionals use is fundamental to providing survivor-centered support because it serves as an indicator of nonjudgmental and affirming services.

DEFINITIONS

Even a cursory examination of the sexual assault literature will reveal a plethora of terms and definitions that highlight the complexity of the language used in this area of the field. For example, Muehlenhard et al. (1992) found that the definitions used by sexual assault scholars differ in numerous ways, including the sexual act described, the parameters of consent, the people involved, and who determines whether or not the incident is considered sexual assault. Thus, even experts in the field use terms and definitions differently, and the confusion can be exacerbated when discussing sexual victimization with laypeople. From an empirical perspective, the specific definitions and questions posed can dramatically impact the demonstrated rate of sexual violence and consequently bias the knowledge base (Bolen & Scannapieco, 1999). From an assessment perspective, clinicians need to be aware that the number and nature of questions used will influence whether or not the client endorses experiencing particular forms of victimization (Hamby &

Koss, 2003). From a service delivery perspective, professionals need to be mindful that they cannot assume that they fully understand how certain terms are being used by others; therefore, they need to ask nonjudgmental, open-ended questions to query any potential disclosures.

In addition to being more aware that the use of language in this area varies widely by both scholars and laypeople, professionals also need to be mindful of the potential impact these differences can have on our understanding of this phenomenon. For example, until 2012, the U.S. Federal Bureau of Investigation (FBI) defined rape as "the carnal knowledge of a female, forcibly and against her will" (U.S. Department of Justice, 2014, p. 1). Therefore, the definition specified that the incident had to involve penile-vaginal penetration, physical force, a female victim, and a male perpetrator (U.S. Department of Justice, 2012). This restricted definition failed to acknowledge the range of victimization experiences that actually exist (e.g., penetration with an object, victims of other genders, perpetrators of other genders, victimization facilitated by incapacitation). Since then, the definition has been revised to define rape as "penetration, no matter how slight, of the vagina or anus with any body part or object, or oral penetration by a sex organ of another person, without the consent of the victim" (U.S. Department of Justice, 2014, p. 1). Furthermore, scholars have a better understanding that a wide range of sexually violent acts (e.g., sexual assault, sexual harassment) increase risk for psychosocial difficulties. Although the field has made large strides in being more inclusive in sexual violence work, there is a lag in knowledge among both providers and the general public about what sexual assault can and does look like. Ultimately, language is powerful in that it creates longstanding constraints for what types of incidents should be considered sexual assault and how we talk about sexual violence.

Professionals should also consider the sociopolitical and cultural factors, such as social power and gender roles, that influence the way we talk about sexual assault. As stated by Hare-Mustin and Maracek, "meaning making and control over language are important resources held by those in power" (1990, p. 25). In a patriarchal society, the language surrounding sexual assault is influenced by the privilege held by heterosexual, cisgender men (Worell & Remer, 1992). For example, men are often given the "benefit of the doubt" in accusations of sexual assault perpetrated against women (Henley & Kramarae, 1991), which is illustrated by male perpetrators who are acquitted because they claim that female victims did not clearly say "no" and lawyers who defend their male clients by discussing the clothing that female victims were wearing at the time of the crime. Another example is that male survivors of sexual assault are largely rendered invisible because of the masculinity rhetoric perpetuated by men toward other men (Turchik & Edwards, 2012), such as the myth that "real men cannot be raped." A consequence of this narrative is that male survivors are often hesitant to seek services or disclose their victimization to potential sources of support. For example, data have suggested that men who screened positive for military sexual trauma were less likely to receive services than women who screened positive for military sexual trauma (Office of Mental Health Services, 2011). When asked about barriers to care following military sexual trauma, male veterans reported concerns related to their masculinity and sexuality, in addition to barriers that are not specific to male survivors (e.g., embarrassment, fear of not being believed, lack of knowledge about available services; Turchik et al., 2013). In sum, professionals need to recognize that people's knowledge and use of particular words and definitions will vary widely and that beliefs engrained in our society (e.g., gender roles, masculinity) create barriers to care for many survivors.

TERMINOLOGY

In addition to considering the influence of how terms such as rape are defined, professionals need to think about the connotations of particular words they may use while delivering services. One example of a set of terms to consider is the use of the word "survivor" versus "victim," which comes into play as an individual conceptualizes what happened to them and forms an identity in the aftermath of victimization (Parker & Mahlstedt, 2010). The term "victim" is often associated with perceptions of the person as weak and powerless and is indicative of lingering negative effects following victimization (Hockett et al., 2014; Thompson, 2000). Conversely, the term "survivor" is often associated with strength, more effective coping strategies, and recovery (Hockett et al., 2014; Thompson, 2000). Overall, individuals who have experienced sexual assault typically perceive the term "survivor" as more positive and less stigmatizing than the term "victim" (Leisenring, 2006; Thompson, 2000). However, it is important to note that this is not universal because some individuals perceive the term "victim" as essential to communicating that a crime occurred (Leisenring, 2006; Thompson, 2000). Overall, best practice would allow survivors the time and opportunity to work through their own meaning making following victimization, and professionals should validate this process by using the language that the survivor decides best represents them and their experience (Hockett & Saucier, 2015).

In general, individuals typically perceive themselves as victims in the immediate aftermath of victimization, but as more time passes, they tend to identify as survivors (Kelly et al., 1996; Thompson, 2000). For this reason, most scholars, including the authors of this book, use the term "victim" when writing about the time period during the crime and the term "survivor" when referencing any time period after the crime. However, from a service delivery perspective, it is important that the disclosure recipient remain neutral (Thompson, 2000). Professionals should serve as a "sounding board" by validating and supporting the person as they explore their own thoughts and feelings about the incident(s) and should not push their own language on the client. Sexual assault survivors have also noted that it is extremely helpful to hear the thoughts of others who have experienced victimization, such as in group therapy or support groups, because it is validating and provides them an opportunity to evaluate their own thoughts (Thompson, 2000). In general, given that the discourse on sexual assault often blames the victim or encourages survivors to stay silent, the act of talking about

Box 2.1

SUMMARY OF KEY RECOMMENDATIONS

Disclosure recipients should remain neutral.

Professionals should serve as a "sounding board" by validating and supporting.

Professionals should not push their own language on the client.

Survivors may find it helpful to hear the thoughts of others who have experienced victimization.

Survivors may feel empowered by talking about sexual assault.

Survivors are "experts on their own experiences."

---

sexual assault in a supportive environment can be empowering to survivors and is increasingly being seen as a form of social activism (Kelly et al., 1996; Leisenring, 2006; Thompson, 2000; Worell & Remer, 1992). Ultimately, survivors are "experts on their own experiences" (Mason & Clemens, 2008, p. 74) and the words professionals use should convey that. See Box 2.1 for a summary of key recommendations.

RAPE ACKNOWLEDGMENT

Professionals also need to be aware that the single word that has been the most problematic related to sexual assault is "rape" (Hamby & Koss, 2003). In fact, only 40% of female rape survivors use the word "rape" to describe their victimization (i.e., acknowledged survivors; Wilson & Miller, 2016). The remaining 60% are considered unacknowledged survivors because they use non-victimizing language, such as "bad sex" or "miscommunication," to describe their victimization (Koss, 1989; Littleton et al., 2007). Although unacknowledged rape is common among all rape survivors, the rates are even higher among male survivors (Reed et al., 2020) and survivors who identify as heterosexual (Wilson & Newins, 2019). Thus, professionals need to be careful when conducting assessments because many of the screening instruments commonly used in clinical practice, such as the Life Events Checklist for DSM-5 (Weathers et al., 2013), contain potentially problematic terms, such as "rape." Clinicians are encouraged to use behaviorally specific language, such as the items on the Sexual Experiences Survey Short Form Victimization (Koss et al., 2007), to better detect unacknowledged rape and sexual assault. More advice related to assessment will be discussed in Chapter 4.

It is also important to know that it is common for survivors to express uncertainty about what happened. For example, they may say they are unsure if the incident should be considered rape or they may blame themselves for what happened. This uncertainty should not be perceived by professionals as reason to question the survivor or to assume the person was not assaulted. Robust research has suggested that how a survivor's rape script (i.e., beliefs about what constitutes "typical" rape) relates to the characteristics of their own assault will impact their conceptualization of the incident (Kahn, 2004). For example, a survivor who believes that rape is typically perpetrated by a stranger who uses physical force will be less likely to acknowledge their own victimization as rape if the perpetrator was an acquaintance and if minimal force was used (Bondurant, 2001). Doubt and self-blame are typical experiences among survivors, and professionals should normalize this reaction and remain neutral sources of support.

Professionals are also encouraged to engage in self-evaluation to consider their own rape scripts and to what extent they hold beliefs consistent with rape myths (Worell & Remer, 1992). Rape myths "affect subjective definitions of what constitutes a 'typical rape', contain problematic assumptions about the likely behavior of perpetrators and victims, and paint a distorted picture of the antecedents and consequences of rape" (Bohner et al., 2009, p. 18). Several studies have found that professionals hold beliefs similar to laypeople, such as victim blaming, particularly toward male survivors or survivors with particular characteristics (e.g., wore a halter top and shorts at the time of the crime, engaged in less resistance, sustained less serious physical injuries; see van der Bruggen & Grubb, 2014, for review). Furthermore, male providers are more likely to believe rape myths than providers of other genders (see van der Bruggen & Grubb, 2014, for review). It is vital that professionals self-monitor because reactions to disclosures have been found to be a function of both the survivor's conceptualization of what happened to them and the disclosure recipient's adherence to rape myths. Specifically, a study found that disclosure recipients who largely rejected rape myths gave survivors affirming and supportive reactions, regardless of the language the survivor used to describe the incident (Wilson et al., 2021). Disclosure recipients who believed rape myths provided less affirming and more negative reactions to the unacknowledged survivor than the acknowledged survivor. Thus, professionals who reject rape myths are better prepared to meet survivors where they are and provide survivor-centered services, regardless of the language the survivor uses to describe their victimization.

Lastly, it is imperative that professionals understand it is not their place to "push" survivors toward being an acknowledged survivor. Although acknowledged rape is associated with greater likelihood of seeking services and reporting the crime, as well as reduced likelihood of revictimization (Littleton et al., 2017; Walsh et al., 2016), some evidence suggests that acknowledged survivors also have greater posttraumatic stress disorder (PTSD) symptoms (Layman et al., 1996; Littleton et al., 2006). It has been posited that unacknowledged rape may be beneficial in the short term because it allows the survivor to perceive the incident as less stressful, which is associated with less psychological distress (Littleton et al., 2009). Then, with time, the survivor may begin to acknowledge the incident as rape, which may be associated with an increase in symptomatology. In light of the mixed evidence regarding the impact of rape acknowledgment on psychosocial functioning, it is recommended that professionals not rush survivors in their recovery process and allow them the time and space to use the language they are most comfortable with as they make meaning of what happened.

CONCLUSION

The language and definitions used in the sexual violence literature create many problems in terms of service delivery. For example, in this chapter, we highlighted some of the issues that arise when using the term "rape." However, other potential terms, such as "sexual assault" and "unwanted sex," have also been shown to be problematic (Cleere & Lynn, 2013; Wilkinson, 2008). This issue is noteworthy because both of these terms are used on common instruments, such as the Life Events Checklist for DSM-5 (Weathers et al., 2013), and are part of everyday language. Research has demonstrated that survivors of sexual assault are no more likely, or perhaps even less likely, to use the term "sexual assault" to label their experience than survivors of rape are to label their experience a "rape" (Cleere & Lynn, 2013). While labeling the event as a sexual assault may convey that the professional views the event as serious, it may also conflict with the survivor's current conceptualization of the event. Conversely, using the phrase "unwanted sex" with a survivor may minimize their victimization experience and imply that the professional takes it less seriously. Ultimately, words matter.

One of the most important objectives for professionals when working with sexual assault survivors is to validate the survivor, and language is one of the most powerful tools for doing so (Worell & Remer, 1992). Professionals should be mindful of the words they choose and carefully consider the ways their words could impact others. It is also recommended that professionals pay close attention to the language the survivors use. The words they choose can convey important information about how they are conceptualizing their victimization (e.g., blaming themselves) and can inform the provider on the language the survivor will be most comfortable with. Similar to best practices for delivering services more generally, professionals should listen more than they speak, ask open-ended questions void of judgment, and reflect back what they hear from clients. When survivors use non-victimizing language or terminology that the professional believes minimizes the severity of the incident, the professional should consider how that choice of language may have been helpful for the survivor in the past, how that language may be helpful for the survivor now, and what, if any, negative impact it is having on the survivor currently. This information can help the professional determine whether to address the label and how to do so. For example, a survivor who is experiencing distress but also minimizing the event may be disappointed in themselves for their current level of functioning, which can lead to self-blame or exacerbate their difficulties. The professional should consider exploring the severity of the event with the survivor and provide validation of the seriousness of the incident, regardless of whether the survivor begins using a different label or not. Given the evidence that talking about sexual assault can be empowering for survivors, professionals should be motivated to help survivors find their own voice and affirm them during their meaning-making process.

REFERENCES

Bohner, G., Eyssel, F., Pina, A., Siebler, F., & Viki, G. T. (2009). Rape myth acceptance: Cognitive, affective and behavioural effects of beliefs that blame the victim and exonerate the perpetrator. In M. Horvath & J. Brown (Eds.), *Rape: Challenging contemporary thinking* (pp. 17–45). Willan.

Bolen, R. M., & Scannapieco, M. (1999). Prevalence of child sexual abuse: A corrective meta-analysis. *Social Science Review, 73*(3), 281–313. https://doi.org/10.1086/514425

Bondurant, B. (2001). University women's acknowledgment of rape: Individual, situational, and social factors. *Violence Against Women, 7*(3), 294–314. https://doi.org/10.1177/1077801201007003004

Cleere, C., & Lynn, S. J. (2013). Acknowledged versus unacknowledged sexual assault among college women. *Journal of Interpersonal Violence, 28*(12), 2593–2611. https://doi.org/10.1177/0886260513479033

Hamby, S. L., & Koss, M. P. (2003). Shades of gray: A qualitative study of terms used in the measured of sexual victimization. *Psychology of Women Quarterly, 27*(3), 243–255. https://doi.org/10.1111%2F1471-6402.00104

Hare-Mustin, R. T., & Maracek, J. (1990). Gender and the meaning of difference: Postmodernism and psychology. In R. T. Hare-Mustin & J. Maracek (Eds.), *Making a difference: Psychology and the construction of gender* (pp. 22–64). Yale University Press.

Henley, N. M., & Kramarae, C. (1991). Gender, power, and miscommunication. In N. Coupland, H. Giles, & J. Wiemann (Eds.), *Miscommunication and problematic talks* (pp. 18–43). Sage.

Hockett, J. M., McGraw, L. K., & Saucier, D. A. (2014). A "rape victim" by any other name: The effects of labels on individuals' rape-related perceptions. In H. Pishwa & R. Schulze (Eds.), *Expression of inequality in interaction: Power, dominance, and status* (pp. 81–104). John Benjamins Publishing Company.

Hockett, J. M., & Saucier, D. A. (2015). A systematic review of "rape victims" versus "rape survivors": Implications for theory, research, and practice. *Aggression and Violent Behavior, 25*(Part A), 1–14. https://doi.org/10.1016/j.avb.2015.07.003

Kahn, A. S. (2004). 2003 Carolyn Sherif award address: What college women do and do not experience as rape. *Psychology of Women Quarterly, 28*(1), 9–15. https://doi.org/10.1111%2Fj.1471-6402.2004.00117.x

Kelly, L., Burton, S., & Regan, L. (1996). Beyond victim or survivor: Sexual violence, identity and feminist theory and practice. In L. Adkins & V. Merchant (Eds.), *Sexualizing the social: Power and the organization of sexuality* (pp. 77–101). St. Martin's Press.

Koss, M. P. (1989). Hidden rape: Sexual aggression and victimization in a national sample of students in higher education. In M. A. Pirog-Good & J. E. Stets (Eds.), *Violence in dating relationships: Emerging social issues* (pp. 145–184). Praeger.

Koss, M. P., Abbey, A., Campbell, R., Cook, S., Norris, J., Testa, M., Ullman, S., West, C., & White, J. (2007). Revising the SES: A collaborative process to improve assessment of sexual aggression and victimization. *Psychology of Women Quarterly, 31*(4), 357–370. https://doi.org/10.1111/j.1471-6402.2007.00385.x

Layman, M. J., Gidycz, C. A., & Lynn, S. J. (1996). Unacknowledged versus acknowledged rape victims: Situational factors and posttraumatic stress. *Journal of Abnormal Psychology, 105*(1), 124–131. https://doi.org/10.1037/0021-843X.105.1.124

Leisenring, A. (2006). Confronting "victim" discourses: The identity work of battered women. *Symbolic Interaction, 29*(3), 307–330. https://doi.org/10.1525/si.2006.29.3.307

Littleton, H. L., Axsom D., & Grills-Taquechel, A. (2009). Sexual assault victims' acknowledgement status and revictimization risk. *Psychology of Women Quarterly, 33*(1), 34–42. https://doi.org/10.1111/j.1471-6402.2008.01472.x

Littleton, H. L., Axsom, D., Radecki Breitkopf, C., & Berenson, A., (2006). Rape acknowledgment status relates to disclosure, coping, worldview, and reactions received from others. *Violence and Victims, 21*(6), 761–778. https://doi.org/10.1891/0886-6708.21.6.761Littleton, H., Grills, A., Layh, M., & Rudolph, K. (2017). Unacknowledged rape and re-victimization risk: Examination of potential mediators. *Psychology of Women Quarterly, 41*(4), 437–450. https://doi.org/10.1177/0361684317720187

Littleton, H. L., Rhatigan, D., & Axsom, D. (2007). Unacknowledged rape: How much do we know about the hidden sexual assault victim? *Journal of Aggression, Maltreatment, and Trauma, 14*(4), 57–74. https://doi.org/10.1300/J146v14n04_04

Mason, S. E., & Clemens, S. E. (2008). Participatory research for rape survivor groups. *Affilia: Journal of Women and Social Work, 23*(1), 66–76. https://doi.org/10.1177%2F0886109907310459

Muehlenhard, C. L., Powch, I.G., Phelps, J. L., & Giusti, L. M. (1992). Definitions of rape: Scientific and political implications. *Journal of Social Issues, 48*(1), 23–44. https://doi.org/10.1111/j.1540-4560.1992.tb01155.x

Office of Mental Health Services. (2011). *Summary of military sexual trauma-related outpatient care, fiscal year 2010.* Department of Veterans Affairs, Office of Mental Health Services.

Parker, J. A., & Mahlstedt, D. (2010). Language, power, and sexual assault: Women's voices on rape and social change. In S. J. Behrens & J. A. Parker (Eds.), *Language in the real world: An introduction to linguistics* (pp. 139–163). Routledge.

Paul, L., Gray, M., Elhai, J. D., & Davis, J. L. (2009). Perception of peer rape myth acceptance and disclosure among college sexual assault survivors. *Psychological Trauma: Theory, Research, Practice, and Policy, 1*(3), 231–241. https://doi.org/10.1037/a0016989

Reed, R. A., Pamlanye, J. T., Truex, H. R., Murphy-Neilson, M. C., Kunaniec, K. P., Newins, A. R., & Wilson, L. C. (2020). Higher rates of unacknowledged rape among men: The role of rape myth acceptance. *Psychology of Men & Masculinities, 21*(1), 162–167. https://doi.org/10.1037/men0000230

Thompson, M. (2000). Life after rape: A chance to speak? *Sexual and Relationship Therapy, 15*(4), 325–343. https://doi.org/10.1080/713697439

Turchik, J. A., & Edwards, K. M. (2012). Myths about male rape: A literature review. *Psychology of Men and Masculinity, 13*(2), 211–226. https://doi.org/10.1037/a0023207

Turchik, J. A., McLean, C., Rafie, S., Hoyt, T., Rosen, C. S., & Kimerling, R. (2013). Perceived barriers to care and provider gender preferences among veteran men who experienced military sexual trauma: A qualitative analysis. *Psychological Services, 10*(2), 213–222. https://doi.org/10.1037/a0029959

U.S. Department of Justice. (2012). *An updated definition of rape*. https://www.justice.gov/archives/opa/blog/updated-definition-rape

U.S. Department of Justice. (2014). *Rape addendum: Uniform crime reporting program changes definition of rape*. https://ucr.fbi.gov/crime-in-the-u.s/2013/crime-in-the-u.s.-2013/rape-addendum/rape_addendum_final.pdf

van der Bruggen, M., & Grubb, A. (2014). A review of the literature relating to rape victim blaming: An analysis of the impact of observer and victim characteristics on attribution of blame in rape cases. *Aggression and Violent Behavior, 19*(5), 523–531. https://doi.org/10.1016/j.avb.2014.07.008

Walsh, K., Zinzow, H. M., Badour, C. L., Ruggiero, K. J., Kilpatrick, D. G., & Resnick, H. S. (2016). Understanding disparities in service seeking following forcible versus drug- or alcohol-facilitated/incapacitated rape. *Journal of Interpersonal Violence, 31*(14), 2475–2491. https://doi.org/10.1177/0886260515576968

Weathers, F. W., Blake, D. D., Schnurr, P. P., Kaloupek, D. G., Marx, B. P., & Keane, T. M. (2013). *The Life Events Checklist for DSM-5 (LEC-5)—Standard*. https://www.ptsd.va.gov/

Wilkinson, C. (2008). *Unwanted sex versus rape: How the language used to describe sexual assault impacts perceptions of perpetrator guilt, victim blaming, and reporting*. Unpublished doctoral dissertation, Indiana University of Pennsylvania.

Wilson, L. C., & Miller, K. E. (2016). Meta-analysis of the prevalence of unacknowledged rape. *Trauma, Violence, & Abuse, 17*(2), 149–159. https://doi.org/10.1177/1524838015576391

Wilson, L. C., & Newins, A. R. (2019). Rape acknowledgment and sexual minority identity: The indirect effect of rape myth acceptance. *Psychology of Sexual Orientation and Gender Diversity, 6*(1), 113–119. https://doi.org/10.1037/sgd0000304

Wilson, L. C., Truex, H. R., Murphy-Neilson, M. C., Kunaniec, K. P., Pamlanye, J. T., & Reed, R. A. (2021). How female disclosure recipients react to women survivors: The impact of rape acknowledgment and rejection of rape myths. *Sex Roles, 84*, 337–346. https://doi.org/10.1007/s11199-020-01169-3

Worell, J., & Remer, P. (1992). *Feminist perspectives in therapy an empowerment model for women*. John Wiley & Sons.

3

The Role of Reactions
to Disclosure in Mental
Health Among Survivors
of Sexual Assault

In the aftermath of sexual assault, survivors often have a range of needs (e.g., medical, emotional, legal), which subsequently leads to a series of decisions. For every need they perceive they have, survivors have to determine whether or not they will disclose their assault to others and in what detail. While receiving services and support may help mitigate the negative mental and physical health consequences of sexual assault, the potential for these benefits is contingent on the responses they receive from other people. Ullman (1996a) noted, "Perhaps the most important factor in real-life disclosures of traumatic events is the recipient of the disclosures who may determine both the type of reaction experienced by victims and the impact of that reaction on the victim" (p. 555).

Social support is multifaceted in that it encompasses perceived support (e.g., an individual's subjective evaluation of the availability and quality of support from those around them), enacted support (e.g., actual support offered and received by others), structural support (e.g., number and degree of availability of others who can offer support), and social reactions (e.g., behaviors that communicate the affect/beliefs of the disclosure recipient; Barrera, 1986; Dworkin et al., 2019; Zalta et al., 2021). Although all of these components of social support are significant predictors of posttraumatic functioning, the largest effect sizes have been demonstrated for social reactions, underscoring the important role of the disclosure recipient (Zalta et al., 2021). Social reactions can range from positive (e.g., providing emotional support) to negative (e.g., not believing the survivor), and one disclosure recipient can provide a blend of positive and negative reactions, even within a single interaction (Dworkin et al., 2019; Ullman, 2010). Negative reactions can be overt and blatant (e.g., victim blaming) or well-meaning but problematic (e.g., asking "Were you drinking?"). Furthermore, negative social reactions can actually be the absence of any response at all (e.g., failure to provide any support after learning about someone's victimization experience; Dworkin et al., 2019; Ullman, 2010). Given that a fear of negative social reactions is the primary reason that sexual assault survivors delay disclosure or fail to disclose their victimization to others (Ullman et al., 2020), this is an important area of self-reflection and potential growth for providers who work with survivors.

In this chapter, we discuss a range of topics related to disclosure by sexual assault survivors. First, we summarize numerous correlates of when and why survivors disclose their assault to others. Although the literature has identified several trends and themes in this area, which we highlight, we do want to note that each individual survivor will make their own decisions regarding disclosing their assault(s) and their particular circumstances may differ from what is discussed here. Second, we summarize the available information on the typical social reactions survivors receive from people in their lives, with an emphasis on formal support sources (e.g., medical and mental health professionals, police). Third, we discuss the psychosocial impact of social reactions on survivors with an eye toward elucidating how professionals may inadvertently harm survivors while delivering services. Finally, in light of the powerful influence professionals can have on survivors' recovery, we make recommendations for ways providers can provide more survivor-centered and affirming services.

WHEN AND WHY SURVIVORS DISCLOSE TO OTHERS

The majority of sexual assault survivors tell at least one person about their victimization, with most survivors telling approximately three individuals (Littleton, 2010; Ullman & Filipas, 2001). It is important to keep in mind that most of the research in this area has been cross-sectional, which means less is known about the temporal process of disclosure across different disclosure recipients. However, the existing literature has demonstrated that most survivors first disclose to an informal source of support, and friends are the most common recipients (Aherns et al., 2007). In particular, female sexual assault survivors tend to first disclose to a female peer (Orchowski & Gidycz, 2012). However, many survivors tell both formal (e.g., medical professional) and informal (e.g., friend) sources of support, and mental health professionals are the most likely formal sources to receive a disclosure (Ullman, 1996b). While approximately one-third of survivors immediately tell someone in their life about their victimization, another third of survivors fear negative reactions and wait several days or weeks, while the remaining third delay disclosing for over a year or may never discuss what happened to them (Filipas & Ullman, 2001; Sudderth, 1998; Ullman et al., 2020; Ullman & Filipas, 2001). Because nondisclosure tends to limit the resources, services, and support available to survivors, it is important to understand what contributes to survivors' decisions regarding if and when they tell others about their victimization. However, professionals also need to consider that nondisclosure may be protective for some individuals (e.g., greater control over their "story," prevention of retaliation from the assailant for telling others about the crime), and survivors should never be pushed to disclose their victimization if they are not ready. However, clinicians should carefully assess the difference between avoidance symptoms of posttraumatic stress disorder (PTSD) and nondisclosure that is protective. Furthermore, mental health professionals need to be prepared to gently guide their clients through discussing difficult details of the trauma, such as during exposure activities. More information about psychotherapy is discussed in Chapter 5.

Survivors disclose their victimization for many reasons, including perceiving that it will be helpful, such as to obtain emotional support or tangible aid, or to pursue justice for their assault. Research suggests that survivors are more likely to disclose sexual assault experiences to providers, including mental health professionals, physicians, police, and rape crisis center staff, if the incident conforms to the "real rape" stereotype. More specifically, if the assault was perpetrated by a stranger, resulted in physical injury, and/or involved fear of death (Ullman & Filipas, 2001), then survivors are more likely to seek services, including legal, medical, and mental health services. It has also been suggested that survivors of more stereotypic rape may disclose to formal sources (e.g., police, physicians) more quickly following the incident than those who experience other types of assault (e.g., perpetrated by known assailant, no physical injury; Golding et al., 1989; Ullman & Filipas, 2001). Research has also shown that survivors who are younger, do not have children, or are Black or Latinx are less likely to disclose their victimization than those who are older, have children, or are White (Aherns et al., 2010; Tillman et al., 2010; Ullman & Filipas, 2001). In addition to these survivor and assault characteristics, research has also found that greater apprehensions about being believed or blamed, traditional beliefs about gender roles and sexuality, concerns about family, fear of burdening others, social expectations to not disclose, and a perceived lack of support are also associated with nondisclosure (Aherns et al., 2010; Ullman et al., 2020). Furthermore, it is likely that numerous cultural factors impact disclosure (e.g., stigma toward seeking mental health services, language barriers, distrust of providers, immigration status; Bryant-Davis et al., 2009; Ullman & Lorenz, 2020). Please see Chapter 9 for more discussion on working with particular populations of sexual assault survivors.

In addition to considering how characteristics of the survivor and assault may impact disclosure decisions, providers should also consider how characteristics of their own profession may impact rates of disclosure. Here, we will focus on aspects of the legal and medical professions. Issues more specific to mental health professionals will be discussed in Chapters 4, 5, 6, 7, and 8. In terms of the legal field, for every 100 rapes committed, 5 to 20 are reported to the police, 0.4 to 5.4 are prosecuted, 0.2 to 4.2 result in a conviction, and only 0.2 to 2.8 result in incarceration (Lonsway & Archambault, 2012). As a result, survivors may be hesitant to disclose to police because they believe that disclosing will not result in any serious consequences for the perpetrator. Furthermore, they may worry that disclosing to the police could upset the perpetrator (if it is someone known to them), which may not seem worth the risk if the likelihood of incarceration is low. In the medical field, most rape survivors who seek medical care are not advised to get a pregnancy test, are not given information on pregnancy prevention (e.g., morning after pill), and are not given information about sexually transmitted diseases (Campbell & Bybee, 1997; National Victim Center, 1992). Furthermore, the intrusive nature of a pelvic exam immediately following a rape is often described as "traumatizing" by survivors (Parrot, 1991). Thus, some of the disciplines that work with sexual assault survivors have a reputation for not providing the desired services or outcomes, or for delivering them in a potentially harmful manner, which can impact the likelihood that a survivor will seek those services. Even when improvements are made at a specific location or facility, fears based on outdated information or information about other facilities may still negatively impact disclosure likelihood. Furthermore, negative experiences with one provider, such as a physician, can impact whether that survivor will tell others about their victimization in the future (Aherns, 2006). Martin and Powell (1994) suggested that these issues arise when an organization or system prioritizes goals that are in conflict with the needs of the sexual assault survivor. For example, a survivor may be seeking validation and support, but an emergency room is focused on treating as many patients as quickly as possible. This difference in goals may ultimately lead the survivor to perceive those providers as uncaring and/or insensitive.

Although we certainly acknowledge that the demands, policies, and financial constraints of particular workplaces and disciplines may make survivor-centered work more challenging, there are several ways organizations can provide survivor-centered care. For example, victim advocates and similar positions (e.g., hospital accompaniment advocates) can be valuable resources for survivors by helping them navigate legal processes and/or medical procedures, while advocating for the needs of the survivor and (typically) serving as a confidential outlet for the survivor. When available, survivors should be informed of the option to have an advocate present and/or to meet with an advocate later. If survivors wish to have an advocate accompany them, agencies should respect these wishes to the extent that it is possible. Additionally, agencies and institutions should ensure that the staff members who interact with sexual assault survivors are adequately trained and possess the necessary skills to effectively and appropriately conduct their job duties. For example, many hospitals do not have any full-time staff members who have completed sexual assault nurse examiner (SANE) training, which is a specialized training that covers the collection of forensic evidence and expert witness testimony, as well as how to interact with survivors in the immediate aftermath of trauma. In these situations, staff may feel unprepared to offer high-quality services to survivors and may ultimately provide substandard care. Therefore, discipline-specific training on how to serve sexual assault survivors is a vital part of offering comprehensive services in any field. Professionals are also encouraged to take the time to carefully explain the steps involved in any procedure or process, communicate realistic expectations for timelines and outcomes, and attend to the emotional needs of survivors. For example, professionals should carefully explain what is involved in a SANE exam and patiently answer all questions prior to starting. They should also explain what will happen with the evidence that is collected, as well as the timeline for the processing of the kit. Staff members should also take the time to provide patient education (e.g., information on pregnancy tests and sexually transmitted diseases) as well as validate and emotionally support the survivor. These are just a few examples, and we encourage all providers to consider ways in which they can modify and improve policies, procedures, and service delivery to make the experience more affirming and supportive of sexual assault survivors.

SOCIAL REACTIONS TOWARD RAPE VICTIMS

Most sexual assault survivors receive both positive and negative social reactions when they disclose their victimization to others (Aherns et al., 2007; Campbell et al., 2001a). Fortunately, survivors tend to receive more positive social reactions than negative social reactions from both informal and formal sources of support (Campbell et al., 2001a; Filipas & Ullman, 2001; Ullman, 1996a). Some of the more common positive reactions include providing tangible support (e.g., resources, advice, information) and emotional support (e.g., empathy, kindness, validation; Aherns et al., 2007; Campbellet al., 2001a). Conversely, negative social reactions tend to include blaming, shaming, distracting, or controlling the survivor (Aherns et al., 2007; Campbell et al., 2001a). Although survivors often agree on the types of reactions they find helpful, there are some individual differences in how survivors perceive particular reactions and responses (Campbell et al., 2001a; Dworkin et al., 2018). For example, there is a lack of agreement among survivors on whether it is helpful or harmful when a disclosure recipient makes decisions for them or tells them to "move on" from what happened to them (Campbell et al., 2001a). Therefore, providers should be aware that a discrete categorical framework of negative and positive reactions is likely oversimplified in terms of real-life disclosure interactions given that there appear to be more nuanced, individual differences in how survivors perceive particular reactions. It is also important to note that it is the survivor's perception of the reaction as harmful or hurtful that predicts mental and physical health and not the reaction itself (Campbell et al., 2001a). Therefore, providers need to be aware that their reactions may be perceived differently by different survivors (Dworkin et al., 2018). In line with this, we recommend that disclosure recipients begin by validating, supporting, and believing the survivor, as there is more consensus among survivors that this type of response is perceived as helpful (Dworkin et al., 2018). Furthermore, disclosure recipients should continue to view and treat the survivor the same as they did before the disclosure rather than treating them as though they are "damaged" or "changed" by what happened to them (Dworkin et al., 2018). Other reactions, such as distracting the survivor, are less consistently perceived as helpful and therefore should be avoided unless a survivor indicates this type of response would be appreciated.

What is particularly troubling is that sexual assault survivors report that they are more likely to receive negative reactions (e.g., egocentric, controlling, victim-blaming reactions) from formal sources of support than informal sources (Aherns et al., 2007; Golding et al., 1989; Ullman, 1996a, 1996b; Ullman & Filipas, 2001). But at the same time, survivors also report that they are more likely to receive some types of positive reactions, such as tangible aid, from providers than family and friends (Ullman & Filipas, 2001). Among providers, rape crisis staff have been reported to be the most helpful, followed by legal professionals, mental health professionals, clergy, physicians, and, lastly, police (Golding et al., 1989; Koon-Magnin & Schulze, 2019). For example, one study found that while 100% of survivors who disclosed to police reported they received tangible aid, more than 70% also reported that the police blamed them for the assault in some way (Koon-Magnin & Schulze, 2019). Therefore, although providers often do provide helpful information and services, it may come at the cost of more harmful reactions. In fact, an entire literature base has been dedicated to this phenomenon, referred to as second injury (Symonds, 1980) or secondary victimization (Campbell et al., 2001b). It is also advised that, after establishing a therapeutic relationship, mental health professionals consider inquiring about the reactions survivors may have received from other sources of support. Assessing reactions to disclosure is important because negative reactions from other individuals, particularly professionals, may contribute to the survivor's difficulties or may impact their willingness to share important details about the incident. It is apparent that professionals still have work to do in order to more effectively promote and support survivor well-being.

PSYCHOSOCIAL IMPACT OF REACTIONS ON SURVIVORS

As mentioned earlier, sexual assault survivors are often motivated to disclose what happened to them because they perceive that it would be beneficial to their recovery in some way. And, in fact, studies have found evidence that positive social reactions are associated with more adaptive coping and greater perceived control among survivors, which is associated with fewer PTSD symptoms (Ullman & Peter-Hagene, 2014). Not surprising, negative social reactions have been linked to greater depression symptoms (Orchowski et al., 2013), PTSD symptoms (Jacques-Tiura et al., 2010; Ullman et al., 2007), alcohol misuse (Peter-Hagene & Ullman, 2014), and distress (Littleton, 2010). And there is preliminary evidence to suggest that negative social reactions may be particularly detrimental for Black survivors (Jacques-Tiura et al., 2010), which will be further discussed in Chapter 9. To elucidate the impact of reactions on functioning, DeCou et al. (2017) demonstrated that negative reactions from others impact survivors' psychological functioning by increasing their shame related to their victimization. Moreover, a longitudinal study demonstrated that negative social reactions did in fact predict PTSD symptoms over time, and PTSD symptoms in turn predicted additional negative social reactions in the future (Ullman & Peter-Hagene, 2016). Finally, a meta-analysis of the literature demonstrated that although positive reactions are associated with fewer psychosocial difficulties among survivors, negative social reactions have a larger impact on survivor functioning (Dworkin et al., 2019). Taken together, the existing body of research points to the powerful influence of negative social reactions, in particular, and indicates that harmful responses may impact how survivors feel about themselves and their assault. Additionally, survivors' psychological functioning may impact the way in which disclosure recipients perceive and respond to them because some difficulties may manifest in a way that makes working with survivors more challenging (e.g., avoidance, feelings of detachment, irritability, or anger). Furthermore, witnessing high levels of distress or hearing about traumatic experiences may overwhelm the disclosure recipient (DePrince et al., 2014). It is particularly problematic that survivors with greater levels of distress may receive more negative reactions because these survivors are the individuals who would arguably benefit the most from services. Ultimately, providers should receive training on typical trauma responses so that they are prepared to deliver competent, evidence-based services to all survivors, regardless of the level of difficulties clients may be experiencing or the severity of the trauma they experienced.

DISCLOSURE RECIPIENT IMPLICATIONS

Although we recognize that each provider will need to identify and navigate discipline-specific policies and issues, several general recommendations apply across fields.

First, because rape myth acceptance is one factor associated with disclosure recipient reactions and how professionals interact with survivors, providers should engage in self-assessment of their beliefs related to rape (Krahe, 2016; Wilson et al., 2021; Worell & Remer, 1992). Survivors report that some of the most common rape myths held by disclosure recipients relate to what the victim was wearing at the time of the crime, why the victim went to the location of the crime (e.g., perpetrator's house), and disbelief that one can be raped by a partner (Filipas & Ullman, 2001). Agencies and institutions are encouraged to provide training specifically geared toward preparing professionals to work with survivors, which should include material on rape myths and sexist beliefs. For example, most mental health professionals report that they do not receive any training during graduate school specific to working with sexual assault survivors and have to seek out that training on their own after graduation (Campbell et al., 1999).

Second, prior research has demonstrated that a trusting relationship between the survivor and disclosure recipient may facilitate more positive reactions from disclosure recipients and/or more understanding by the survivor if the disclosure recipient should inadvertently respond negatively (Dworkin et al., 2018). Therefore, consistent with substantial literature, rapport is extremely important when working with sexual assault survivors and providers should receive adequate training in this skillset.

Third, given that survivors often perceive helpers as insensitive or uncaring because the priorities of the system in which they work are inconsistent with the needs of the survivor, it is important that providers assess for the needs of the survivor. Additionally, agencies and providers should be explicit and upfront about what services they can provide and be prepared to offer referrals when they are not the appropriate resource given the needs of the survivor.

Fourth, providers are encouraged to take the time to validate survivors and convey empathy during the course of service delivery. As Stenius and Veysey (2005) articulate, it is more about *how* services are delivered than the services themselves.

Fifth, as was mentioned earlier, providers should be well versed in PTSD symptoms and trauma-related difficulties, and the necessary training should be provided to them (Gagnon et al., 2018).

Finally, professionals should be mindful of the way in which survivors' interactions with other formal sources of support may impact their own service delivery (Campbell et al., 1999). For example, survivors' symptoms may ebb and flow in reaction to aspects of the legal process. Because of this, it is beneficial for mental health professionals to be knowledgeable about the legal process as well as common issues stemming from other individuals to whom survivors may disclose (e.g., medical professionals, family members).

We further discuss issues related to assessment and psychotherapy in Chapters 4 and 5, and we provide case examples in Chapters 6, 7, and 8 to illustrate ways in which these topics can be addressed.

CONCLUSION

Although the literature has disproportionately focused on how survivor and assault characteristics relate to long-term functioning, a growing body of literature has suggested that a sociocultural framework may be more informative for understanding outcomes following sexual assault (e.g., Neville & Heppner, 1999; Ullman, 1999). This perspective is consistent with the meta-analytic evidence that has demonstrated that a lack of social support, particularly receiving negative social reactions, is one of the most robust risk factors for posttraumatic difficulties (Brewin et al., 2000; Dworkin et al., 2019; Ozer et al., 2003; Zalta et al., 2021). Given that one negative social reaction can outweigh the potential benefit of positive social reactions (Campbell et al., 2009) and formal sources of support seem to be more likely than informal source to engage in harmful responses (e.g., victim blaming; Aherns et al., 2007; Golding et al., 1989; Ullman, 1996a, 1996b; Ullman & Filipas, 2001), we see this as a high-priority area of improvement for professionals who work with sexual assault survivors. We are by no means stating or implying that all, or even the majority of, providers engage in problematic interactions with sexual assault survivors. Instead, we aim (1) to minimize the potential for a survivor to receive a response from a provider that is perceived as harmful and (2) to promote survivors' access to helpful and supportive formal sources of support.

REFERENCES

Aherns, C. E. (2006). Being silenced: The impact of negative social reactions on the disclosure of rape. *American Journal of Community Psychology, 38*(3–4), 263–274. https://doi.org/10.1007/s10464-006-9069-9

Aherns, C. E., Campbell, R., Ternier-Thames, N. K., Wasco, S. M., & Sefl, T. (2007). Deciding whom to tell: Expectations and outcomes of rape survivors' first disclosures. *Psychology of Women Quarterly, 31*(1), 38–49. https://doi.org/10.1111/j.1471-6402.2007.00329.x

Aherns, C. E., Rios-Mandel, L. C., Isas, L., & del Carmen Lopez, M. (2010). Talking about interpersonal violence: Cultural influences on Latinas' identification and disclosure of sexual assault and intimate partner violence. *Psychological Trauma, 2*(4), 284–295. https://doi.org/10.1037/a0018605

Barrera, M. (1986). Distinctions between social support concepts, measures, and models. *American Journal of Community Psychology, 14*(4), 413–445. https://doi.org/10.1007/BF00922627

Brewin, C. R., Andrews, B., & Valentine, J. D. (2000). Meta-analysis of risk factors for posttraumatic stress disorder in trauma-exposed adults. *Journal of Counseling and Clinical Psychology, 68*(5), 748–766. https://doi.org/10.1037//0022-006X.68.5.748

Bryant-Davis, T., Chung, H., & Tillman, S. (2009). From the margins to the center: Ethnic minority women and the mental health effects of sexual assault. *Trauma, Violence, and Abuse, 10*(4), 330–357. https://doi.org/10.1177/1524838009339755

Campbell, R., Ahrens, C. E., Sefl, T., Wasco, S. M., & Barnes, H. E. (2001a). Social reactions to rape victims: Healing and hurtful effects on psychological and physical health outcomes. *Violence and Victims, 16*(3), 287–302. https://doi.org/10.1891/0886-6708.16.3.287

Campbell, R., & Bybee, D. (1997). Emergency medical services for rape victims: Detecting the cracks in service delivery. *Women's Health: Research on Gender, Behavior, and Policy, 3*(2), 75–101.

Campbell, R., Dworkin, E., & Cabral, G. (2009). An ecological model of the impact of sexual assault on women's mental health. *Trauma, Violence, & Abuse, 10*(3), 225–246. https://doi.org/10.1177/1524838009334456.

Campbell, R., Raja, S., & Grining, P. L. (1999). Training mental health professionals on violence against women. *Journal of Interpersonal Violence, 14*(10), 1003–1012. https://doi.org/10.1177%2F088626099014010001

Campbell, R., Wasco, S. M., Aherns, C. E., Sefl, T., & Barnes, H. E. (2001b). Preventing the "second rape": Rape survivors' experiences with community service providers. *Journal of Interpersonal Violence, 16*(12), 1239–1259. https://doi.org/10.1177/088626001016012002

DeCou, C. R., Cole, T. T., Lynch, S. M., Wong, M. M., & Matthews, K. C. (2017). Assault-related shame mediates the association between negative social reactions to disclosure of sexual assault and psychological distress. *Psychological Trauma: Theory, Research, Practice, and Policy, 9*(2), 166–172. https://doi.org/10.1037/tra0000186

DePrince, A. P., Welton-Mitchell, C., & Srinivas, T. (2014). Longitudinal predictors of women's experiences of social reactions following intimate partner abuse. *Journal of Interpersonal Violence, 29*(13), 2509–2523. https://doi.org/10.1177/0886260513520469

Dworkin, E. R., Brill, C. D., & Ullman, S. E. (2019). Social reactions to disclosure of interpersonal violence and psychopathology: A systematic review and meta-analysis. *Clinical Psychology Review, 72*, Article 101750. https://doi.org/10.1016/j.cpr.2019.101750

Dworkin, E. R., Newton, E., & Allen, N. E. (2018). Seeing roses in the thorn bush: Sexual assault survivors' perceptions of social reactions. *Psychology of Violence, 8*(1), 100–109. https://doi.org/10.1037/vio0000082

Filipas, H. H., & Ullman, S. E. (2001). Social reactions to sexual assault victims from various support sources. *Violence and Victims, 16*(6), 673–692.

Gagnon, K. L., Wright, N., Srinivas, T., & DePrince, A. P. (2018). Survivors' advice to service providers: How to best serve survivors of sexual assault. *Journal of Aggression, Maltreatment, & Trauma, 27*(10), 1125–1144. https://doi.org/10.1080/10926771.2018.1426069

Golding, J. M., Siegel, J. M., Sorenson, S. B., Burnam, M. A., & Stein, J. A. (1989). Social support sources following sexual assault. *Journal of Community Psychology, 17*(1), 92–107. https://doi.org/10.1002/1520-6629(198901)17:1<92::AID-JCOP2290170110>3.0.CO;2-E

Jacques-Tiura, A. J., Tkatch, R., Abbey, A., & Wegner, R. (2010). Disclosure of sexual assault: Characteristics and implications for posttraumatic stress symptoms among African American and Caucasian survivors. *Journal of Trauma & Dissociation, 11*(2), 174–192. https://doi.org/10.1080/15299730903502938

Koon-Magnin, S., & Schulze, C. (2019). Providing and receiving sexual assault disclosures: Findings from a sexually diverse sample of young adults. *Journal of Interpersonal Violence, 34*(2), 416–441. https://doi.org/10.1177/0886260516641280

Krahe, B. (2016). Societal responses to sexual violence against women: Rape myths and the "real rape" stereotype. In H. King, S. Redo, & E. Shea (Eds.), *Women and children as victims and offenders: Background, prevention, reintegration: Suggestions for succeeding generations* (pp. 671–700). Springer International Publishing.

Littleton, H. L. (2010). The impact of social support and negative disclosure reactions on sexual assault victims: A cross-sectional and longitudinal investigation. *Journal of Trauma & Dissociation, 11*(2), 210–227. https://doi.org/10.1080/15299730903502946

Lonsway, K. A., & Archambault, J. (2012). The "justice gap" for sexual assault cases: Future directions for research and reform. *Violence Against Women, 18*(2), 145–168. https://doi.org/10.1177/1077801212440017

Martin, P., & Powell, R. (1994). Accounting for the "second assault": Legal organizations framing of rape victims. *Law and Social Inquiry, 19*(4), 853–890. https://doi.org/10.1111/j.1747-4469.1994.tb00942.x

National Victim Center. (1992). *Rape in America: A report to the nation.*

Neville, H. A., & Heppner, M. J. (1999). Contextualizing rape: Reviewing sequelae and proposing a culturally inclusive ecological model of sexual assault recovery. *Applied and Preventive Psychology, 8*(1), 41–62.

Orchowski, L. M., & Gidycz, C. A. (2012). To whom do college women confide following sexual assault? A prospective study of predictors of sexual assault disclosure and social reactions. *Violence Against Women, 18*(3), 264–288. https://doi.org/10.1177/1077801212442917

Orchowski, L. M., Untied, A. S., & Gidycz, C. A. (2013). Social reactions to disclosure of sexual victimization and adjustment among survivors of sexual assault. *Journal of Interpersonal Violence*, *28*(10), 2005–2023. https://doi.org/10.1177/0886260512471085

Ozer, E. J., Best, S. R., Lipsey, T. L., & Weiss, D. S. (2003). Predictors of posttraumatic stress disorder and symptoms in adults: A meta-analysis. *Psychological Bulletin*, *129*(1), 52–73. https://doi.org/10.1037/0033-2909.129.1.52

Parrot, A. (1991). Medical community response to acquaintance rape: Recommendations. In L. Bechhofer & A. Parrot (Eds.), *Acquaintance rape: The hidden victim* (pp. 304–316). Wiley.

Peter-Hagene, L. C., & Ullman, S. E. (2014). Social reactions to sexual assault disclosure and problem drinking: Mediating effects of perceived control and PTSD. *Journal of Interpersonal Violence*, *29*(8), 1418–1437. https://doi.org/10.1177/0886260513507137

Stenius, V. M. K., & Veysey, B. M. (2005). "It's the little things": Women, trauma, and strategies for healing. *Journal of Interpersonal Violence*, *20*(10), 1155–1174. https://doi.org/10.1177/0886260505278533

Sudderth, L. K. (1998). "It'll come right back at me": The interactional context of discussing rape with others. *Violence Against Women*, *4*(5), 572–594. https://doi.org/10.1177/1077801298004005004

Symonds, M. (1980). The "second injury" to victims. *Evaluation and Change*, 36–38. https://doi.org/10.1057/ajp.2009.38

Tillman, S., Bryant-Davis, T., Smith, K., & Marks, A. (2010). Shattering silence: Exploring barriers to disclosure for African American sexual assault survivors. *Trauma, Violence, & Abuse*, *11*(2), 59–70. https://doi.org/10.1177/1524838010363717

Ullman, S. E. (1996a). Correlates and consequences of adult sexual assault disclosure. *Journal of Interpersonal Violence*, *11*(4), 554–571. https://doi.org/10.1177/088626096011004007

Ullman, S. E. (1996b). Do social reactions to sexual assault victims vary by support provider? *Violence and Victims*, *11*(2), 143–156. https://doi.org/10.1891/0886-6708.11.2.143

Ullman, S. E. (1999). Social support and recovery from sexual assault: A review. *Aggression and Violent Behavior: A Review Journal*, *4*(3), 343–358. https://doi.org/10.1016/S1359-1789(98)00006-8

Ullman, S. E. (2010). *Talking about sexual assault: Society's response to survivors.* American Psychological Association.

Ullman, S. E., & Filipas, H. H. (2001). Correlates of formal and informal support seeking in sexual assaults victims. *Journal of Interpersonal Violence*, *16*(10), 1028–1047. https://doi.org/10.1177/088626001016010004

Ullman, S. E., Filipas, H. H., Townsend, S. M., & Starzynski, L. L. (2007). Psychosocial correlates of PTSD symptom severity in sexual assault survivors. *Journal of Traumatic Stress*, *20*(5), 821–831. https://doi.org/10.1002/jts.20290

Ullman, S. E., & Lorenz, K. (2020). African American sexual assault survivors and mental health help-seeking: A mixed methods study. *Violence Against Women*, *26*(15-16), 1941–1965. https://doi.org/10.1177/1077801219892650

Ullman, S. E., O'Callaghan, E., Shepp, V., & Harris, C. (2020). Reasons for and experiences of sexual assault nondisclosure in a diverse community sample. *Journal of Family Violence, 35,* 839–851. https://doi.org/10.1007/s10896-020-00141-9

Ullman, S. E., & Peter-Hagene, L. (2014). Social reactions to sexual assault disclosure, coping, perceived control and PTSD symptoms in sexual assault survivors. *Journal of Community Psychology, 42*(4), 495–508. https://doi.org/10.1002/jcop.21624

Ullman, S. E., & Peter-Hagene, L. (2016). Longitudinal relationships of social reactions, PTSD, and revictimization in sexual assault survivors. *Journal of Interpersonal Violence, 31*(6), 1074–1094. https://doi.org/10.1177/0886260514564069

Wilson, L. C., Truex, H. R., Murphy-Neilson, M. C., Kunaniec, K. P., Pamlanye, J. T., & Reed, R. A. (2021). How female disclosure recipients react to women survivors: The impact of rape acknowledgment and rejection of rape myths. *Sex Roles, 84,* 337–346. https://doi.org/10.1007/s11199-020-01169-3

Worell, J., & Remer, P. (1992). *Feminist perspectives in therapy: An empowerment model for women.* John Wiley & Sons.

Zalta, A. K., Tirone, V., Orlowska, D., Blais, R. K., Lofgreen, A., Klassen, B., Held, P., Stevens, N. R., Adkins, E., & Dent, A. L. (2021). Examining moderators of the relationship between social support and self-reported PTSD symptoms: A meta-analysis. *Psychological Bulletin, 147*(1), 33–54. http://dx.doi.org/10.1037/bul0000316

4

Assessing Sexual Assault and Reacting to Client Disclosures During Assessment

Regardless of the reason a client is presenting to a mental health provider, the relationship begins with an assessment of some sort. Given the high rates of sexual assault and the subsequent serious mental health sequelae, nearly all mental health providers will work with survivors of sexual assault at some point in time, whether the provider is aware of the client's victimization history or not. Therefore, it is important that mental health providers be aware of assessment options and how language used during assessment may affect the likelihood that a client who experienced a sexual assault will disclose their victimization. As discussed in Chapter 2, many survivors of sexual assault do not label their experience as "rape" or "sexual assault," which presents challenges when assessing for a history of sexual assault.

In this chapter, we discuss the importance of wording in both self-report and clinician-administered measures. While a variety of assessment measures are reviewed, given the number of assessment measures available and the fact that new assessment measures are developed regularly, this chapter is not intended to discuss all available instruments. Rather, this chapter focuses on identifying benefits and drawbacks of wording used in common measures to help clinicians select an appropriate existing instrument and/or generate their own questions for intake paperwork and assessment interviews.

ASSESSMENT OF SEXUAL ASSAULT AMONG ADULTS

The "gold standard" self-report assessment measures of sexual assault are the victimization versions of the Sexual Experiences Survey (SES; Koss et al., 2007). The SES uses behaviorally specific questions to assess unwanted sexual touching, attempted and completed oral sexual activity, attempted and completed vaginal penetration, and attempted and completed anal penetration via various perpetration strategies. The SES–Short Form Victimization (SES-SFV) asks participants about five perpetration strategies—two involve verbal coercion, one involves incapacitation, and two involve physical force, physical violence, and threats of physical force. A strength of the SES is the use of behaviorally specific wording and avoidance of terms such as *sexual assault* and *rape* until the final item. This wording is advantageous because it does not require participants to label their experience in any specific way in order to endorse the item. Another strength of the SES is the inclusion of a wide range of perpetration strategies, including verbal coercion. While verbal coercion to compel an individual to engage in sexual activity does not meet most legal and research definitions of rape, survivors of sexual coercion are also at risk for negative psychological outcomes (e.g., Brown et al., 2009; de Visser et al., 2007). Therefore, assessment of sexual coercion can also be important in clinical practice and research.

While research with women supports reliability and validity of the information gathered from the SES (Johnson et al., 2017), research examining reliability and validity in a sample of men revealed mixed findings, including low test–retest reliability for coercion experiences (Anderson et al., 2018). Additionally, a primary limitation of the SES is that the questions regarding vaginal and anal penetration are worded such that the victim must have experienced penetration of the vagina or anus; therefore, if a man was forced to penetrate another individual's vagina or anus, this experience would not be captured by the SES. As a result, some researchers have modified the SES to use more neutral wording on these items to allow the victim to have been penetrated or to have been forced to penetrate (e.g., Littleton et al., 2020). As a result, while the SES has many strengths, there are some limitations to its use, particularly with men.

While the SES is commonly used in research on sexual assault, it is less commonly used in clinical settings because clinicians often need to assess for a history of multiple types of potentially traumatic events, making lengthy questionnaires focused on one specific trauma type unfeasible for many providers. There are numerous measures that assess trauma exposure in adults (see Elhai et al., 2005; and Gray & Slagle, 2006, for reviews). A few of the most common self-report measures of trauma exposure in clinical settings are the Traumatic Life Events Questionnaire (TLEQ; Kubany et al., 2000), the Life Events Checklist for the *Diagnostic and Statistical Manual of Mental Disorders*, 5th edition (LEC-5; Weathers et al., 2013b), and the Stressful Life Events Screening Questionnaire (Goodman et al., 1998). Each of these measures contains at least two questions designed to assess history of sexual assault, as do most measures of general trauma exposure.[1] There is variability across measures in terms of the type(s) of unwanted sexual contact assessed and the wording used to describe lack of consent. Specifically, some questions ask about sexual touching, others ask about intercourse, and still others use the term "sexual assault." Some measures include a "catch-all" item to assess

---

1. However, some assessment measures focused on specific types of trauma exposure, such as those designed to assess combat exposure, do not assess experiences of sexual assault.

unwanted sexual experiences not covered by other items. Regarding the concept of nonconsent, measures vary in whether they specify that the act was completed without consent, whether they indicate physical force or threats of physical force needed to be used, and whether they include other ways in which an individual may have been unable to consent (e.g., intoxication).

In terms of clinical interviews, many diagnostic interviews, such as the Anxiety and Related Disorders Interview Schedule for DSM-5 (ADIS-5; Brown & Barlow, 2014), the Diagnostic Interview for Anxiety, Mood, and OCD and Related Neuropsychiatric Disorders (DIAMOND; Tolin et al., 2013), and the Structured Clinical Interview for DSM-5 Disorders, Clinician Version (SCID-5-CV; First et al., 2016), that assess posttraumatic stress disorder (PTSD) as part of the battery include screening questions regarding trauma exposure. The questions typically inquire about "sexual assault" or "sexual violence." While questions sometimes include childhood sexual abuse, the questions do not typically define consent (or lack of consent) or the types of sexual contact that are included. In contrast, interviews specifically designed for PTSD, including the Clinician Administered PTSD Scale for DSM-5 (CAPS-5; Weathers et al., 2013a) and PTSD Symptom Scale—Interview for DSM-5 (PSS-I-5; Foa et al., 2016), typically encourage use of a screening measure for potentially traumatic events prior to the interview and then obtain a brief description of the previously identified event as part of the interview.

As can be seen in this discussion, many assessment measures for trauma exposure in adults use terms such as *sexual assault* or *sexual violence* without providing definitions or clarifications. Therefore, many of these assessments require clients to label their experience as a sexual assault and are open to interpretation by the client. Furthermore, the term *sexual violence* may also not be endorsed by some participants, particularly if their assault did not involve physical violence. As a result, clinicians should be aware that some of these measures may not detect some instances of sexual assault, depending on how the client labels and conceptualizes their experience or how they interpret the question. Clinicians who wish to assess a broader range of unwanted sexual experiences may want to consider providing behaviorally specific definitions or asking about a broader range of unwanted sexual experiences in their intake questionnaires and during their intake interviews. Furthermore, if the clinician detects any hesitancy or uncertainty from the client, the clinician should ask further questions to ensure clients have ample opportunity to disclose their victimization if they choose.

ASSESSMENT OF SEXUAL ABUSE AND SEXUAL ASSAULT AMONG CHILDREN AND ADOLESCENTS

Numerous screening measures for trauma exposure in children are available (see Eklund et al., 2018; Strand et al., 2005, for reviews). Many screening measures have both child and caregiver report versions, such as the Child and Adolescent Trauma Screen (CATS; Sachser et al., 2017) and the Child Trauma Screen (CTS;

Lang & Connell, 2017), and there are also interviews to assess trauma exposure, such as the Children's PTSD Inventory (Saigh et al., 2000). The wording used to assess child sexual abuse in these measures varies greatly. For example, some measures inquire whether children have been made to "do sexual things" and others ask whether anyone has touched private or sexual parts of the child's body or whether the child has been made to touch someone else's private or sexual body parts. Some measures, such as the CTS, avoid using the term "sex" by asking about touching of "parts of your body that a bathing suit covers." Furthermore, measures vary in whether the child needed to feel uncomfortable during the incident(s) or if they were unable to consent.

Similar to the discussion about measures for adults, clinicians should be aware that the wording of the assessment measures they use to assess exposure to potentially traumatic events will affect some clients' responses and therefore clinicians' abilities to detect exposure to sexual abuse and sexual assault. For children and adolescents, it is particularly important to consider the client's developmental level and social history when assessing unwanted sexual contact. Specifically, how to best word items and refer to sexual contact will depend on the child's developmental level. Additionally, when children begin dating, relationship violence can then occur, which results in increased possibilities for incidents, such as coercion and rape by an acquaintance or romantic partner, to occur. Furthermore, the relevance of consent in determining whether sexual abuse or sexual assault occurred varies by the developmental level of the child and the age of the perpetrator. Because of the wide range of experiences that could meet criteria for sexual abuse or sexual assault among children, it is difficult to balance keeping assessment procedures as brief as possible while also being thorough. In fact, some measures of trauma exposure in adults (e.g., the TLEQ) contain multiple questions to separately assess child abuse events (e.g., sexual contact that occurs by an older individual or sexual contact without consent before adolescence) from adolescent sexual assault due to the differences in how these incidents occur.

In addition to finding measures with wording the clinician believes is appropriate for assessing unwanted sexual experiences among children and adolescents in their setting, clinicians must consider whether to obtain information from the child, a caregiver, multiple caregivers, or a combination. Clinicians should consider the developmental level of the child in making this decision. When possible, gathering information from the child (potentially in combination with gathering information from caregiver[s]) is encouraged, as children may not have disclosed incidents of unwanted sexual contact to their caregivers and it is possible that a caregiver could be a perpetrator, which may lead to nondisclosure by a caregiver.

REACTING TO DISCLOSURES OF SEXUAL ASSAULT DURING ASSESSMENTS

Whether a client discloses experiencing a sexual assault on a screening question, during a clinical interview, during an interview assessing psychosocial history, or any other part of the assessment, the clinician's reaction to the disclosure is particularly important. Clinician reactions will convey information to the client about how the clinician conceptualizes the client's report, which will likely impact the client's willingness to share further information about their unwanted sexual experience and possibly other clinically relevant information.

First and foremost, when discussing the sexual assault with the client during the assessment, the clinician should use the client's language for labeling the experience. Given that many survivors do not use labels such as rape and sexual assault to label their experience, if the clinician uses these labels when the client does not use them, the client may believe the clinician does not understand what they are reporting. Furthermore, as discussed in Chapter 2, the available research evidence is inconsistent in terms of whether acknowledgment leads to better mental health outcomes among survivors. Additionally, during the assessment phase, it is unlikely that the clinician will have the time to conduct a nuanced discussion regarding labels for unwanted sexual experiences that may allow for sufficient psychoeducation to help clients reconsider their labels.

Second, clinicians need to be aware that their reactions to disclosures may convey information to the client about the clinician's ability to "handle" the disclosure. Some clients have reported that when they disclosed to a previous clinician, the clinician cried, changed the topic, or made comments such as, "I would never be able to handle it if that happened to me." These clients note that these reactions caused them to not talk about the sexual assault any further, which interfered with their ability to receive the treatment they needed to address their trauma symptoms. Some clients who indicated their previous clinician made initial comments about how horrific the event was or about how the clinician could not have handled such an experience said they believed the clinician meant well but still noted that these reactions led to them not wanting to discuss the issue further.

Third, clinicians should be aware that some clients react negatively to statements such as, "I know that these experiences are very difficult." Some clients note that unless the clinician has also experienced a sexual assault, they cannot possibly "know" how difficult the experience is to handle. Therefore, clinicians need to be mindful of balancing how they display empathy without accidentally indicating that they fully understand the client's experience.

Fourth, reactions can convey clinician's opinions about sexual assault, including any rape myths they endorse. While many clinicians know to avoid questions such as, "What were you wearing?" they may ask other questions that suggest, or have the potential to be perceived as suggesting, victim blaming. For example, clinicians may want to determine the client's ability to consent and ask about the client's substance use prior to the sexual assault. This information may be necessary to obtain for assessment purposes (e.g., determining if Criterion A for PTSD is met) or treatment purposes (e.g., challenging self-blame cognitions, gathering information for exposure therapy), but it is important for clinicians to consider when they ask these questions and how they phrase them. It may also be helpful for clinicians to explain why they are asking these questions.

Fifth, clinicians should carefully consider how much information they need about the unwanted sexual experience before asking for additional information. For example, clinicians may need a brief description of the event to determine if it meets Criterion A for PTSD, but a detailed description of the incident is not necessary for this purpose. In contrast, the unwanted sexual experience may not be particularly relevant to some clients' presenting concerns, making details even less important. While most survivors can share a general description of their unwanted sexual experience without undue distress, sharing more detailed information may be distressing, particularly for clients with PTSD and significant re-experiencing symptoms. It can be helpful to tell clients prior to asking follow-up questions regarding the unwanted sexual experience that clients do not need to provide a great deal of details. Many survivors felt out of control during the sexual assault, so it is important to allow them to control the level of detail and the pace at which they share during the assessment phase.

Sixth, clinicians need to ensure that they do not assume clients have a specific diagnosis (e.g., PTSD) or need trauma-focused treatment simply because they have experienced a sexual assault. While it is important to assess how traumatic events have affected the client, many individuals are resilient following traumatic events (Bonanno, 2005). Furthermore, even if a client has some mental health symptoms as a result of an unwanted sexual experience, these symptoms may not be the client's primary presenting problem or concern.

CONCLUSION

In sum, the prevalence of unwanted sexual experiences almost guarantees that clinicians will work with individuals who have had an unwanted sexual experience. Furthermore, media coverage of sexual assaults often involves promotion of rape myths and victim blaming, and many survivors receive negative reactions to disclosures of sexual assault. As a result, it is imperative that clinicians be prepared to handle client disclosures during assessments competently. Clinicians must carefully evaluate screening measures or interview questions used to assess history of sexual abuse and unwanted sexual experiences, particularly if they want to maximize the likelihood of detecting these experiencing among their clients. Furthermore, clinicians need to learn to respond to disclosures in a way that is supportive of the survivor, does not reinforce rape myths or victim blaming, and provides the survivor control over the level of disclosure.

REFERENCES

Anderson, R. E., Cahill, S. P., & Delahanty, D. L. (2018). The psychometric properties of the Sexual Experiences Survey–Short Form Victimization (SES-SFV) and characteristics of sexual victimization experiences in college men. *Psychology of Men & Masculinity*, 19(1), 25–34. https://doi.org/10.1037/men0000073

Bonanno, G. A. (2005). Resilience in the face of potential trauma. *Current Directions in Psychological Science, 14*(3), 135–138. https://doi.org/10.1111/j.0963-7214.2005.00347.x

Brown, A. L., Testa, M., & Messman-Moore, T. L. (2009). Psychological consequences of sexual victimization resulting from force, incapacitation, or verbal coercion. *Violence Against Women, 15*(8), 898–919. https://doi.org/10.1177/1077801209335491

Brown, T. A., & Barlow, D. H. (2014). *Anxiety and Related Disorders Interview Schedule for DSM-5: Client interview schedule.* Oxford University Press.

de Visser, R. O., Rissel, C. E., Richters, J., & Smith, A. M. A. (2007). The impact of sexual coercion on psychological, physical, and sexual well-being in a representative sample of Australian women. *Archives of Sexual Behavior, 36*(5), 676–686. https://doi.org/10.1007/s10508-006-9129-0

Eklund, K., Rossen, E., Koriakin, T., Chafouleas, S. M., & Resnick, C. (2018). A systematic review of trauma screening measures for children and adolescents. *School Psychology Quarterly, 33*(1), 30–43. https://doi.org/10.1037/spq0000244

Elhai, J. D., Gray, M. J., Kashdan, T. B., & Franklin, C. L. (2005). Which instruments are most commonly used to assess traumatic event exposure and posttraumatic effects?: A survey of traumatic stress professionals. *Journal of Traumatic Stress, 18*(5), 541–545. https://doi.org/10.1002/jts.20062

First, M. B., Williams, J. B., Karg, R. S., & Spitzer, R. L. (2016). *Structured Clinical Interview for DSM-5 Disorders: Clinician version.* American Psychiatric Association.

Foa, E. B., McLean, C. P., Zang, Y., Zhong, J., Rauch, S., Porter, K., Knowles, K., Powers, M. B., & Kauffman, B. Y. (2016). Psychometric properties of the Posttraumatic Stress Disorder Symptom Scale Interview for DSM-5. *Psychological Assessment, 28*(10), 1159–1165. https://doi.org/10.1037/pas0000259

Goodman, L. A., Corcoran, C., Turner, K., Yuan, N., & Green, B. L. (1998). Assessing traumatic event exposure: General issues and preliminary findings for the Stressful Life Events Screening Questionnaire. *Journal of Traumatic Stress, 11*(3), 521–542. https://doi.org/10.1023/A:1024456713321

Gray, M. J., & Slagle, D. M. (2006). Selecting a potentially traumatic event screening measure. *Journal of Trauma Practice, 5*(2), 1–19. https://doi.org/10.1300/J189v05n02_01

Johnson, S. M., Murphy, M. J., & Gidycz, C. A. (2017). Reliability and validity of the Sexual Experiences Survey–Short Form Victimization and Perpetration. *Violence and Victims, 32*(1), 78–92. https://doi.org/10.1891/0886-6708.VV-D-15-00110

Koss, M. P., Abbey, A., Campbell, R., Cook, S., Norris, J., Testa, M., Ullman, S., West, C., & White, J. (2007). Revising the SES: A collaborative process to improve assessment of sexual aggression and victimization. *Psychology of Women Quarterly, 31*(4), 357–370. https://doi.org/10.1111/j.1471-6402.2007.00385.x

Kubany, E. S., Leisen, M. B., Kaplan, A. S., Watson, S. B., Haynes, S. N., Owens, J. A., & Burns, K. (2000). Development and preliminary validation of a brief broad-spectrum measure of trauma exposure: The Traumatic Life Events Questionnaire. *Psychological Assessment, 12*(2), 210–224. https://doi.org/10.1037/1040-3590.12.2.210

Lang, J. M., & Connell, C. M. (2017). Development and validation of a brief trauma screening measure for children: The Child Trauma Screen. *Psychological Trauma: Theory, Research, Practice, and Policy, 9*(3), 390–398. https://doi.org/10.1037/tra0000235

Littleton, H., Downs, E., & Rudolph, K. (2020). The sexual victimization experiences of men attending college: A mixed methods investigation. *Sex Roles, 83*, 595–608. https://doi.org/10.1007/s11199-020-01133-1

Sachser, C., Berliner, L., Holt, T., Jensen, T. K., Jangbluth, N., Risch, E., Rosner, R., & Goldbeck, L. (2017). International development and psychometric properties of the Child and Adolescent Trauma Screen (CATS). *Journal of Affective Disorders, 210*, 189–195. https://doi.org/10.1016/j.jad.2016.12.040

Saigh, P. A., Yasik, A. E., Oberfield, R. A., Green, B. L., Halamandaris, P. V., Rubenstein, H., Nester, J., Resko, J., Hetz, B., & McHugh, M. (2000). The Children's PTSD Inventory: Development and reliability. *Journal of Traumatic Stress, 13*(3), 369–380. https://doi.org/10.1023/A:1007750021626

Strand, V. C., Sarmiento, T. L., & Pasquale, L. E. (2005). Assessment and screening tools for trauma in children and adolescents: A review. *Trauma, Violence, & Abuse, 6*(1), 55–78. https://doi.org/10.1177/1524838004274559

Tolin, D. F., Wootton, B. M., Bowe, W., Bragdon, L., Davis, E., Gilliam, C., Hannan, S., Hallion, L. S., Springer, K., Steinman, S. A., & Worden, B. (2013). *Diagnostic Interview for Anxiety, Mood, and OCD and Related Disorders (DIAMOND)*. Institute of Living/Hartford HealthCare Corporation.

Weathers, F. W., Blake, D. D., Schnurr, P. P., Kaloupek, D. G., Marx, B. P., & Keane, T. M. (2013a). *The Clinician-Administered PTSD Scale for DSM-5 (CAPS-5)*. https://www.ptsd.va.gov/professional/assessment/adult-int/caps.asp

Weathers, F. W., Blake, D. D., Schnurr, P. P., Kaloupek, D. G., Marx, B. P., & Keane, T. M. (2013b). *The Life Events Checklist for DSM-5 (LEC-5)*. https://www.ptsd.va.gov/professional/assessment/te-measures/life_events_checklist.asp

5

Psychotherapy with Sexual Assault Survivors

Issues Related to Disclosure

Because sexual assault is so prevalent, all clinicians need to be prepared to work with survivors of sexual assault, as many survivors who seek services from mental health providers will be looking for treatment. Survivors of sexual assault are at increased risk of a wide range of psychological disorders compared to individuals who have not experienced a sexual assault, with particularly strong effects for posttraumatic stress disorder (PTSD) and depressive disorders (Dworkin, 2020; Dworkin et al., 2017). Given the broad range of psychological disorders associated with sexual assault, clinicians should not assume that a client who discloses a sexual assault during the intake assessment or course of treatment will need PTSD treatment. As discussed in the last chapter, clinicians must conduct thorough intake evaluations to determine which disorder or disorders best fit a survivor's presenting symptoms. Then, the clinician must determine a treatment protocol to best fit the client's current needs based on the clinician's case conceptualization.

In this chapter, we provide recommendations for clinicians using cognitive-behavioral treatments with survivors of sexual assault. The chapter begins with a brief overview of treatments available for various disorders that may develop following sexual assault. However, this overview is not exhaustive, and it is not meant to describe any treatments in detail. Clinicians are encouraged to refer to treatment manuals and attend trainings for specifics about how to implement various treatment protocols. Furthermore, this chapter does not include content on other treatment approaches that may be deemed appropriate for some clients, such as psychopharmacological interventions. This chapter focuses on discussing how clinicians can address disclosure of information about sexual assault during treatment by providing recommendations for exposure therapy, cognitive therapy, and other issues in therapy.

TREATMENTS FOR ADULT SURVIVORS
OF SEXUAL ASSAULT

In general, cognitive-behavioral therapy (CBT) has been shown to be effective for the treatment of PTSD in adults (Guideline Development Panel for the Treatment of PTSD in Adults, 2017; Management of Posttraumatic Stress Disorder Workgroup, 2017). Specific treatment protocols with research support include Prolonged Exposure (PE; Foa et al., 2019), Cognitive Processing Therapy (CPT; Resick et al., 2017), and Trauma Management Therapy (TMT; Beidel et al., 2017). Both PE and TMT involve exposure therapy for PTSD. Specifically, both treatments involve imaginal exposure to the trauma memory, in which the participant repeatedly recalls the traumatic event, and in vivo exposure to trauma reminders and situations that elicit hypervigilance. While there are some differences in how exposure is conducted in the two treatments (e.g., how long each exposure session lasts, whether emotional processing follows imaginal exposure, whether imaginal exposure is assigned as homework), the primary difference between the two treatments is that TMT also includes a skills training component, typically conducted in a group setting, that teaches brief behavioral activation, anger management, sleep hygiene, and social reintegration skills. In contrast, CPT focuses on helping patients use cognitive restructuring skills to address thoughts related to self-blame and in five core areas of safety, trust, control, esteem, and intimacy. Because research to date has not identified factors to predict which patients do best in which treatment, clinicians should consider their level of competence in providing these various treatments, the client's preferences regarding treatment, and the clinician's case conceptualization regarding factors maintaining the client's PTSD symptoms when choosing a treatment protocol.

For clients who present with PTSD and substance use disorders, cognitive-behavioral treatment options include Concurrent Treatment of PTSD and Substance Use Disorders Using Prolonged Exposure (COPE; Back et al., 2015), which combines PE and relapse prevention strategies for substance use, and Seeking Safety (Najavits, 2002), which focuses on teaching skills to increase safe coping strategies. Clients who present with a depressive disorder, an anxiety disorder, or a combination of these disorders (including comorbid alcohol use problems) may benefit from the Unified Protocol for Transdiagnostic Treatment of Emotional Disorders (Barlow et al., 2017; Barlow & Farchione, 2018). Furthermore, a wide range of other treatment protocols for various disorders is available as part of the Oxford University Press's *Treatments That Work* series. In choosing a treatment, clinicians should consider the client's presenting problems and primary diagnosis, as well as the clinician's case conceptualization of factors maintaining psychological symptoms at the time that the client presents to treatment. In particular, it is important that clinicians do not assume trauma-focused treatment for PTSD is required for all survivors of sexual assault. However, given that avoidance is a symptom of PTSD, clinicians must be prepared to determine when avoidance is impacting a survivor's presentation and treatment preferences.

Conversely, the clinician may determine that a survivor's symptoms indicate non–trauma-focused treatment is a better fit for the presenting problem, either because of the primary symptoms or because of the patient's readiness for trauma-focused treatment.

TREATMENTS FOR CHILD SURVIVORS OF SEXUAL ABUSE

The gold-standard treatment of PTSD in children is Trauma-Focused Cognitive Behavioral Therapy (TF-CBT; Cohen et al., 2017). This treatment involves a trauma narrative, which is a form of exposure to the trauma memory, and in vivo exposure to trauma reminders and situations. The treatment also involves training in cognitive restructuring. Furthermore, there is a component focused on increasing safety to reduce the likelihood of future exposure to traumatic events, when it is deemed appropriate by the clinician; for children who experienced child sexual abuse, this component is particularly important to identify ways to reduce the likelihood the child will experience further sexual abuse and other types of abuse. Finally, parent or caregiver involvement is important in TF-CBT so the parent can assist with skills training and exposure.

Alternatively, PE has been adapted for adolescents (Foa et al., 2008). For children with disorders other than PTSD following sexual abuse, the Unified Protocols for Transdiagnostic Treatment of Emotional Disorders in Children and Adolescents (Ehrenreich-May et al., 2018) and other specific manuals are available in the Oxford University Press's *Treatments That Work* series.

CONSIDERATIONS FOR EXPOSURE THERAPY

As noted earlier, exposure therapy for PTSD typically involves both imaginal exposure and in vivo exposure. For both of these components, clinicians must be prepared for clients to disclose additional details of their sexual assault. As noted in Chapter 3, failure to appropriately respond to the additional details disclosed could interfere with the clinician's ability to maximize the effectiveness of exposure therapy.

In imaginal exposure therapy, clients repeatedly recount the memory of the traumatic event that bothers them the most. Regardless of trauma type, clinicians who conduct exposure therapy for PTSD need to be prepared to hear about their clients' traumatic events in detail. Importantly, in order for imaginal exposure to be as effective as possible, clients should include as many details as possible in their narrative in order to increase immersion in the trauma memory. Therefore, clinicians should ensure they have self-care plans in place to help them manage their own reactions to hearing the details of these horrific events.

There are additional considerations that are important for clinicians who use imaginal exposure therapy with survivors of sexual assault. First, talking about sexual behaviors and using sexual terms is generally taboo in everyday conversations. However, clinicians will need to model comfort with discussing these topics and using these terms for the client. In particular, clinicians cannot shy away from asking for additional details about sexual acts and sexual contact. Many clients will attempt to "gloss over" details of the actual sexual assault as a form of avoidance, and it is the clinician's responsibility to ensure the client provides sufficient detail for exposure. For example, the clinician will need to use anatomical terms (e.g., vagina, penis, anus, breast) in these questions. When clinicians show anxiety, discomfort, or timidness when discussing sexual activity, clients are likely to be shy in sharing details of what occurred.

Second, clinicians must be careful to not react in ways that support myths about sexual assault when hearing the details of clients' victimization. Many clients' stories will include details that are not consistent with common stereotypes about rape (e.g., the perpetrator was an acquaintance or romantic partner, no weapon was used). Additionally, clients may have engaged in behaviors that are consistent with victim-blaming rape myths (e.g., dressed provocatively, voluntarily consumed alcohol prior to the assault, voluntarily went to the perpetrator's home). It is also important to consider that some victims of sexual assault experience arousal, and even orgasm, during the incident due to physiological reactions. Clinicians may unintentionally reveal endorsements of stereotypes and myths about sexual assault in their reactions to client disclosures of these details. Even subtle verbal (e.g., "Oh") or nonverbal (e.g., making a face) reactions that suggest surprise can communicate to clients that the clinician doubts their account, questions whether their incident is a sexual assault or rape, or believes that the assault was their fault. How clinicians word follow-up questions is also important. For example, if a client reveals they drank alcohol prior to the sexual assault and the clinician asks, "But you didn't drink enough to become incapacitated, right?" that could send the client messages about whether the clinician considers the event to be serious/traumatic and whether the clinician blames the survivor for the assault.

Third, clinicians should be prepared to hear slang and aggressive terms for body parts and sexual acts. While clinicians can encourage clients to use anatomically correct terms and more generally accepted terms for sexual acts when describing their sexual assault, it is possible that the perpetrator(s), victim, or others used slang terms in dialog during the sexual assault, which may be necessary to include in the trauma narrative used in imaginal exposure. If clinicians demonstrate reluctance to hear this language, clients may worry that the clinician cannot handle hearing their full story and may withhold important details.

In vivo exposure for PTSD typically involves exposure, in real life, to trauma reminders and situations that elicit hypervigilance. In order to design appropriate in vivo exposure activities, clinicians need to create a list of the reminders and situations clients fear and avoid due to their traumatic event (commonly called an exposure hierarchy). When constructing this list, clinicians will need to obtain details about the sexual assault in order to identify trauma reminders to be considered for the exposure hierarchy. For example, clients may report experiencing anxiety when they hear a song that was playing in the perpetrator's bedroom during the sexual assault. As noted earlier, it is important that clinicians attempt to avoid responses that support rape myths during these discussions (e.g., asking the client why they went into the perpetrator's bedroom) or inadvertently communicate disbelief or victim blaming.

CONSIDERATIONS FOR COGNITIVE THERAPY

Cognitive therapy for PTSD involves identifying the client's maladaptive thoughts that resulted from the traumatic experience and are causing problems in the client's life by leading to intense negative emotions and maladaptive thoughts. Clinicians teach clients how to examine their thoughts and change them to be more adaptive. In CPT, a specific cognitive therapy for PTSD, thoughts in the areas of self-blame, safety, trust, control, esteem, and intimacy are emphasized for cognitive restructuring. Clinician reactions to disclosure of details and clinician use of questions during cognitive therapy are critical to ensuring clients do not receive confirmation of maladaptive beliefs during treatment.

First, self-blame is common among survivors of sexual assault. As a result, clinicians conducting cognitive therapy with survivors of sexual assault will likely need to help clients challenge thoughts related to their level of responsibility for the sexual assault. It is important for clinicians to remember that perpetrators bear full responsibility for sexual assault, regardless of the circumstances surrounding the incident, and while there are strategies individuals can use to reduce their risk of victimization, failure to use these strategies does not reduce the perpetrator's level of responsibility or shift responsibility to the patient. Clients often identify multiple reasons they believe they are to blame for the sexual assault (e.g., consuming substances prior to the incident, going to the location where the assault occurred, separating from friends), and it is important that clinicians help clients recognize that these actions (or inactions) do not mean the client was "asking for" sexual assault. While clinicians will likely need to ask probing questions to help clients recognize that these behaviors do not make the client responsible for the sexual assault, clinicians should be careful to explain the cognitive model to clients and the general rationale for asking questions to explore the client's thoughts, take care when wording challenging questions, and be willing to explain the rationale for specific questions if the client reacts negatively to a question. For example, if it seems that the survivor had no reason to suspect that going to the perpetrator's house would lead to a sexual assault, a clinician may ask a client why they decided to go to the perpetrator's home on the night of the sexual assault in an effort to help the client recognize that they did not believe they would be sexually assaulted when they made that decision. However, some clients may perceive that question as the clinician blaming them for the sexual assault. If the clinician notices the client becoming distressed or withdrawing following a question like this, the clinician should ask the client about their reaction, apologize for any errors in wording or tone the clinician may have made, and explain why they asked the question. Furthermore, as noted in Chapter 3, it is vital to establish a strong working relationship with the client prior to beginning therapy because it can help clinicians navigate any misunderstanding (e.g., client misunderstanding the purpose of a question).

Related to the concept of self-blame, survivors who experienced immobility (i.e., a "freeze" response) and those who experienced arousal or orgasm during the assault may report self-blame or confusion related to these reactions. Clinicians must be willing to hear about these reactions from their clients and also be prepared to challenge self-recriminating thoughts without supporting any rape myths. Clinicians should be prepared to discuss the physiological basis of the freeze response and/or arousal and orgasm during sexual assault. In particular, it is very important that clinicians not react with surprise or disbelief that these types of experiences can occur during sexual assault.

If a client disclosed their sexual assault to others prior to treatment, the client may have experienced social reactions that contributed to self-blame and/or concerns about safety and trust. For example, others may have implied that the survivor was to blame for the sexual assault, may have suggested that sexual assault happens because the world is an unsafe place, or may have indicated that others cannot be trusted because sexual assault is a constant threat. When conducting cognitive therapy with survivors of sexual assault, clinicians should be sure to inquire about sources of information for evidence that supports maladaptive cognitions and be willing to hear about negative reactions to disclosures. Additionally, clinicians may need to help clients make sense of negative reactions they may have received from friends, family members, the police, and others. As an example, statements that blame victims for their sexual assault may be a way for others to help protect themselves from feeling vulnerable to sexual assault (e.g., if the victim did something to cause the sexual assault, then the disclosure recipient can protect themself from sexual assault by not engaging in those behaviors).

When challenging thoughts in the areas of esteem and intimacy, clients may reveal negative thoughts regarding body image, self-worth, and sexual intimacy. Clinicians need to be willing to discuss these topics with clients in order to address the client's maladaptive thoughts across domains. Clients may endorse beliefs about being "dirty" or "bad" because they were forced to engage in various sexual acts, and clinicians may need to manage their reactions when hearing about sexual acts that may not fit with the clinician's values and beliefs. Furthermore, some clients may report confusion about their sexuality following a sexual assault. In particular, men who experienced arousal or orgasm due to physiological reasons during the sexual assault may question their sexuality. Clinicians need to understand possible physiological reactions during sexual assault in order to be adequately prepared to help clients examine these thoughts.

Finally, while cognitive therapies for PTSD often do not involve trauma narratives, written trauma narratives are included in some cognitive therapies (e.g., CPT with the trauma account [CPT+A]; Resick et al., 2017). When a trauma account is included in the treatment plan, the same considerations noted earlier for exposure therapy apply.

OTHER CONSIDERATIONS FOR TREATMENT

Even if survivors have not received negative reactions, they may be hesitant to disclose their sexual assault to others, including police, medical personnel, and their social support network. From a cognitive perspective, clinicians can help clients identify the thoughts underlying their reluctance to disclose and evaluate those thoughts. However, clinicians should be particularly careful to take an unbiased, exploratory approach when evaluating these thoughts and make sure they treat clients as the expert on their own lives rather than trying to guide clients toward a decision to disclose. Additionally, clinicians can consider using problem-solving strategies or considering pros and cons of disclosing versus not disclosing to help clients make the best decision for themselves.

Patients, both those who have experienced a sexual assault themselves and those who have not, may disclose during treatment that they have received a disclosure from a friend, family member, or other acquaintance. In discussing this information, clinicians should be careful to not endorse any rape myths, particularly because the clinician's reactions could influence the client's willingness to disclose other information in future sessions or could impact the way the client treats the individual who disclosed to them. Furthermore, clinicians should help patients identify ways they can provide positive responses to the survivor while also respecting the client's own boundaries and protecting the client's mental health.

Clinicians should also be mindful that some clients may be resistant to beginning CBT. One of the most common concerns expressed by trauma survivors is that engaging in a trauma-focused treatment will worsen their symptoms or exceed their ability to cope (Hundt et al., 2015). Discussing the rationale behind CBT may alleviate some of the anxiety related to engaging in this type of psychotherapy. Additionally, engaging the client in the process of selecting an evidence-based treatment, vocalizing confidence that the client can successfully complete the treatment protocol, explaining the steps involved in the treatment protocol, and providing evidence of prior successes based on both research and other clients' testimonials have been found to increase client buy-in (Hundt et al., 2015). Ultimately, given the effectiveness of CBT in alleviating posttrauma difficulties, it is essential that clinicians take the necessary steps to reduce barriers to care.

CONCLUSION

When providing trauma-focused therapy to survivors of sexual assault, clinicians will be exposed to further details than were provided in the initial assessment, regardless of whether a full, detailed trauma narrative is obtained. Clinician reactions to these details will affect clients' willingness to share further details and may impact whether or not they seek additional services from a range of professionals (e.g., whether or not they report the crime to authorities). Furthermore, clinician reactions can serve to either contradict clients' maladaptive cognitions (e.g., empathetic, validating responses can provide evidence against beliefs that survivors will be rejected or judged negatively if they share their experience) or confirm negative beliefs (e.g., showing surprise if a survivor discloses experiencing arousal during the sexual assault). Furthermore, clinicians must model openness to discussing sexual activity in order to allow survivors to fully share the details of their assault and the impact the sexual assault has had on their lives.

REFERENCES

Back, S. E., Foa, E. B., Killeen, T. K., Mills, K. L., Teesson, M., Cotton, B. D., Carroll, K. M., & Brady, K. T. (2015). *Concurrent treatment of PTSD and substance use disorders using Prolonged Exposure (COPE)—Therapist guide*. Oxford University Press.

Barlow, D. H., & Farchione, T. J. (Eds.). (2018). *Applications of the Unified Protocol for Transdiagnostic Treatment of Emotional Disorders*. Oxford University Press.

Barlow, D. H., Farchione, T. J., Sauer-Zavala, S., Latin, H. M., Ellard, K. K., Bullis, J. R., Bentley, K. H., Boettcher, H. T., & Cassiello-Robbins, C. (2017). *Unified Protocol for Transdiagnostic Treatment of Emotional Disorders—Therapist guide* (2nd ed.). Oxford University Press.

Beidel, D. C., Stout, J. W., Neer, S. M., Frueh, B. C., & Lejuez, C. (2017). An intensive outpatient treatment program for combat-related PTSD: Trauma Management Therapy. *Bulletin of the Menninger Clinic, 81*(2), 107–122. doi:10.1521/bumc.2017.81.2.107

Cohen, J. A., Mannarino, A. P., & Deblinger, E. (2017). *Treating trauma and traumatic grief in children and adolescents* (2nd ed.). Guilford Press.

Dworkin, E. R. (2020). Risk for mental disorders associated with sexual assault: A meta-analysis. *Trauma, Violence, & Abuse, 21*(5), 1011–1028. https://doi.org/10.1177/1524838018813198

Dworkin, E. R., Menon, S. V., Bystrynski, J., & Allen, N. E. (2017). Sexual assault victimization and psychopathology: A review and meta-analysis. *Clinical Psychology Review, 56*, 65–81. doi:10.1016/j.cpr.2017.06.002

Ehrenreich-May, J., Kennedy, S. M., Sherman, J. A., Bilek, E. L., Buzzella, B. A., Bennett, S. M., & Barlow, D. H. (2018). *Unified Protocols for Transdiagnostic Treatment of Emotional Disorders in children and adolescents*. Oxford University Press.

Foa, E. B., Chrestman, K. R., & Gilboa-Schechtman, E. (2008). *Prolonged Exposure therapy for adolescents with PTSD: Emotional processing of traumatic experiences: Therapist guide*. Oxford University Press.

Foa, E. B., Hembree, E. A., Rothbaum, B. O., & Rauch, S. A. M. (2019). *Prolonged Exposure therapy for PTSD: Emotional processing of traumatic experiences: Therapist guide* (2nd ed.). Oxford University Press.

Guideline Development Panel for the Treatment of PTSD in Adults. (2017). *Clinical practice guideline for the treatment of posttraumatic stress disorder (PTSD) in adults*. American Psychological Association. https://www.apa.org/ptsd-guideline/ptsd.pdf

Hundt, N. E., Mott, J. M., Miles, S. R., Arney, J., Cully, J. A., & Stanley, M. A. (2015). Veterans' perspectives on initiating evidence-based psychotherapy for posttraumatic stress disorder. *Psychological Trauma: Theory, Research, Practice, and Policy, 7*(6), 539–546. https://doi.org/10.1037/tra0000035

Management of Posttraumatic Stress Disorder Workgroup. (2017). *VA/DOD clinical practice guideline for the management of posttraumatic stress disorder and acute stress disorder*. Department of Veterans Affairs and Department of Defense.

Najavits, L. M. (2002). *Seeking safety: A treatment manual for PTSD and substance abuse*. Guilford Press.

Resick, P. A., Monson, C. M., & Chard, K. M. (2017). *Cognitive Processing Therapy for PTSD: A comprehensive manual*. Guilford Press.

6

Case Example 1

Assessing Sexual Assault

In Chapter 4, we provided recommendations for handling disclosures of sexual assault during assessments. In this chapter, we present a case example of a disclosure that occurs during an intake evaluation. The goal of this chapter is to provide some examples of how a clinician may respond to the disclosure and discuss ways to address various difficulties that could arise in the course of these discussions.

This case example covers an intake assessment with Gabby, a 22-year-old female college student presenting for treatment of depression (note: pseudonyms were used for all case examples and identifying details were changed to protect confidentiality). As part of the intake self-report assessment battery, Gabby completed the Life Events Checklist for DSM-5 (LEC-5) and indicated she had experienced an "other unwanted or uncomfortable sexual experience" (Weathers et al., 2013). Prior to meeting with Gabby, the clinician reviewed the intake questionnaires and noticed this endorsement. Additionally, the clinician noted Gabby scored in the severe range on a measure of depressive symptoms. After obtaining written and verbal consent to conduct the intake assessment, the clinician began by asking about Gabby's presenting concerns.

> *Clinician:* Gabby, thank you again for coming in today to talk with me. To start our discussion today, I'd like to hear what is bringing you in to see me. In other words, what caused you to seek mental health treatment at this time?
>
> *Gabby:* Well, I've been feeling pretty down and sad for a while now. And I just don't feel up to doing anything anymore. I've been missing classes because I just can't seem to get myself out of bed to go to class. I'm worried that my grades are going to be affected if I miss any more classes.
>
> *C:* So, these feelings of sadness have been affecting your attendance in school, which made you want to get treatment before your grades decline?
>
> *G:* Yeah.
>
> *C:* When did you first notice these feelings of sadness?

G: I guess about six months ago.

C: When these feelings started six months ago, was that the first time in your life that you've felt like this or have there been other times in the past that you've felt really sad or down?

G: When I was a junior in high school, my grandmother died, and I remember feeling really sad then. It lasted for a few weeks, and I still feel sad when I think about how much I miss her. But aside from that, I've never felt sad like this before.

C: That's really helpful for me to know. So, about six months ago, you started feeling really down and sad. What has the sadness "looked like" since then?

G: What do you mean?

C: That's a great question. I'm wondering if the sadness has stayed at a constant level since it started six months ago, if it's gotten better, if it's gotten worse, or if it's been a bit up and down.

G: Oh, well, I guess I'd have to say it's been getting worse. When it first started, I thought it would go away, but the past month or so, I don't want to go out with my friends anymore, and I just want to spend all my time in bed.

In this first portion of the assessment, the clinician was focused on gathering information about why the client is coming in for treatment. Furthermore, the clinician learned about the course of the primary symptoms the client is most bothered by at this time. While it would likely be good to assess history of depressive symptoms again when more specific information about various symptoms of depressive disorders is obtained, based on the information the clinician has obtained at this point, it seems that this is the client's first episode of significant depressive symptoms.

Next, the clinician conducted a risk assessment for risk of harm to self and others. Gabby indicated she has never been hospitalized for psychiatric reasons, attempted suicide, engaged in self-injurious behaviors, or thought about suicide. Furthermore, Gabby stated she has not engaged in aggressive behaviors toward others and never had thoughts of killing another person. Following the risk assessment, the clinician inquired about a history of traumatic or stressful events.

C: Next, I want to ask if you have ever experienced any events that you found very stressful or difficult? Or any events or experiences that bothered you a lot or caused changes in your behavior?

G: Like I mentioned before, I felt really sad when my grandmother died seven years ago. I was really close with her.

C: It sounds like your grandmother was a very special person to you. It can be very difficult to lose people we love. What about other stressful or bothersome events or experiences?

G: Nothing else I can think of.

C: OK. Just to make sure I don't miss anything, I noticed on one of the forms you filled out that you indicated you had an uncomfortable or unwanted sexual experience. Is that something that you still think about or still bothers you?

G: Oh, that. Well, I don't like to talk about it. It was just a big mistake on my end.

C: OK. We don't need to talk about it very much right now. But I would like to get a few more details. I don't need specifics at this point, and if I ask anything you don't want to share right now, just let me know. Is that OK with you?

G: I guess.

C: When did this experience occur?

G: About seven months ago.

C: As I mentioned before, I don't need a detailed description right now, but it would really help for me to know just a bit about what happened.

G: There's this guy in one of my classes that I've been talking to. I think he's really hot and nice, so when he invited me over to watch a movie at his house, I was so excited. At that point, I didn't really drink very often, but he had some rum and diet soda, so I drank it. I ended up feeling pretty tipsy, and we made out for a little while. I wanted to stop there, but he kept going. I said "no" and that I didn't want to have sex, but I was too tipsy to leave, so he ended up having sex with me. I really shouldn't have let myself get into that situation.

C: I really appreciate you sharing that information with me today. That sounds like a difficult situation to navigate—wanting him to stop and also thinking that you can't leave. Have you talked to anyone else about what happened that night?

G: I told my best friend about it. She told me I should be happy because it shows he must really like me.

C: I imagine that may have been confusing for her to tell you to be happy about a situation you found uncomfortable or unwanted.

G: Yeah. I haven't told anyone else . . . well, at least not until today when I told you.

In the preceding exchange, we would like to note four specific points. First, it is not uncommon for survivors of sexual assault to omit this event when discussing their history of traumatic or stressful events. In this case, the clinician had information from the self-report battery that conflicted with the client saying her only stressful life event was the death of her grandmother. Some clinicians worry that asking about discrepancies across reporting formats could rupture rapport, which they are trying to build during the initial sessions. However, by not asking about discrepancies, clinicians can miss important information that can lead to challenges in creating a coherent case conceptualization at the conclusion of the intake due to conflicting information. While clinicians should examine possible discrepancies in reporting, they should not assume that failure to disclose an event endorsed on a measure of trauma exposure is intentional or is due to the client trying to avoid talking about the event. For example, Gabby could have responded to the clinician's initial inquiry about the unwanted sexual experience with, "Oh yeah. There was this one time freshman year that a guy went further than I wanted him to, and it bothered me at first, but I haven't thought about that in over a year. I don't think it's had a big impact on me." In that case, if Gabby's presentation of the information seemed genuine, the clinician likely would not need to explore the incident further at this time, as the event was not temporally linked to the onset of symptoms and the client is indicating she does not believe the event had a significant impact on her.

Second, during the intake evaluation, it is typically not necessary to obtain detailed information about traumatic events, including sexual assault. Clinicians need to obtain enough information to determine if the event is relevant to the case conceptualization, and for a diagnosis of posttraumatic stress disorder (PTSD), they need to know if Criterion A is met. However, some patients find describing the event in detail difficult and distressing. Because the clinician likely will not have time to allow the client to fully experience and cope with significant distress during the intake evaluation, it is important for the clinician to emphasize that detailed information is not needed at this stage.

Third, in this example, Gabby does not use the term sexual assault to label her experience on the LEC-5 or during the interview. Instead, it seems she has not acknowledged the sexual assault. As discussed previously, clinicians should not push clients to label their experience in a specific way, particularly during the intake process. The clinician may choose to explore the label later during treatment, particularly since Gabby views the event as her "mistake." If the clinician attempts to change this label during the intake, it could limit rapport building, as clients may not be ready to change their view of the event or may not be willing to discuss the event to that degree, and it could cause the intake evaluation to be drawn out, which would delay starting treatment.

Fourth, toward the end of this discussion, the clinician obtained important information about social reactions to disclosure that may have impacted the client. Specifically, Gabby shared that she told her best friend about the event, and from the description of the interaction, the friend did not view the experience as concerning and minimized the incident. It is likely that this reaction contributed to Gabby not viewing the event as a sexual assault and blaming herself for the event and her reactions, which may be a topic to discuss further in treatment.

The clinician then conducted an assessment of psychosocial history and a structured clinical interview to determine current diagnoses. At the end of the intake, the clinician determined that Gabby had been experiencing a major depressive episode, severe, for the past six months. Gabby did not endorse any reexperiencing or avoidance symptoms of PTSD; however, the clinician believed Gabby's unwanted sexual experience, particularly her self-blame for the event, contributed to her symptoms of depression. At the conclusion of the intake, the clinician presented this conceptualization to Gabby.

C: Now that we've completed the intake evaluation, I'd like to share my thoughts on the results of the assessment.

G: OK.

C: Because you talked about experiencing depressed mood, loss of interest in activities such as going to class and spending time with friends, sleeping too much, weight gain and increased appetite, feeling worthless and guilty, and trouble making decisions, you meet criteria for what we call major depressive disorder.

G: I heard about that in one of my psychology courses. I don't remember much about it, but I have been experiencing all those things, so I guess it fits.

C: OK, I'm glad to hear the diagnosis makes sense to you, and I'd like to provide more information about what I think has contributed to your depression. One thing that seems to have contributed to your depression is that uncomfortable sexual experience from about seven months ago. It seems like it wasn't long after that when these symptoms began, particularly since that is when you said you started to think the experience was your fault. Given this, I'd like us to talk about how to use some of the skills we're going to work on in treatment to address some of your thoughts about that event. What do you think about this?

G: Before I came here, I never thought about how that night affected me, but what you're saying makes sense, I guess. So, we can try it.

In this portion of the assessment, the clinician presented the case conceptualization. Because the clinician believes the sexual assault contributed to Gabby's depression, this hypothesis is discussed. Importantly, the clinician still continued to use language Gabby has already used to describe her experience rather than applying a label of sexual assault. The clinician was also careful about the wording they used when pointing out that Gabby seemed to be blaming herself, which was important for the clinician to avoid inadvertently endorsing any rape myths or appearing as though they thought Gabby was indeed to blame. Furthermore, the clinician offered hope to the client by indicating that there are skills the clinician plans to teach in treatment to help the client address her symptoms and the impact of the sexual assault.

CONCLUSION

In this chapter, we presented portions of an intake evaluation with Gabby, a collegiate woman presenting with depression. These excerpts demonstrate how to address discrepancies in reporting or a client's hesitancy to discuss sexual assault, the importance of establishing the timeline of traumatic events and symptom onset, ways to use the client's language to describe unacknowledged sexual assault, the need to be careful with wording and questions so as not to accidentally endorse rape myths, and how to present a conceptualization that encourages clients to address mental health symptoms secondary to sexual assault.

REFERENCE

Weathers, F. W., Blake, D. D., Schnurr, P. P., Kaloupek, D. G., Marx, B. P., & Keane, T. M. (2013). *The Life Events Checklist for DSM-5 (LEC-5)*. https://www.ptsd.va.gov/professional/assessment/te-measures/life_events_checklist.asp

7

Case Example 2

Unanticipated Disclosures

In Chapters 4 and 5, we discussed recommendations for addressing disclosures of sexual assault during assessment and treatment. In Chapter 6, we presented a case example in which a clinician handled disclosure of a sexual assault during an intake evaluation. While clinicians may be prepared for a disclosure during the intake evaluation when they are gathering information about a new patient, survivors may also disclose a sexual assault at times that the clinician is not expecting it. In this chapter, we present two brief case examples in which a client discloses when the clinician was not expecting the client to do so. The goal of this chapter is to demonstrate ways a clinician might respond to unexpected disclosures and to provide suggestions for how to handle difficulties that may arise in these situations.

EXAMPLE 1

In this first example, the clinician was completing an intake evaluation with an adult man, Damon, who presented for treatment of symptoms of obsessive-compulsive disorder (OCD; note: pseudonyms were used for all case examples and identifying details were changed to protect confidentiality). On the intake questionnaires, when asked if he had experienced any traumatic events, Damon wrote, "N/A." After obtaining informed consent, the clinician began to administer a semistructured interview to assess psychosocial history. When asked about presenting concerns, Damon disclosed that he is worried about losing his job because he arrives 30 to 60 minutes late to work each day due to checking compulsions. He noted he experiences frequent obsessive thoughts involving doubt about whether he locked doors and turned off appliances at home. The clinician then asked about a history of traumatic events.

> *Clinician:* Now that I have an understanding of why you're coming in for treatment, I'd like to get some background information about you and

your life. At any point in time, have you experienced any traumatic events, such as events in which you were worried about your physical safety, saw someone else be killed or in great physical danger, experienced a sexual assault, or were exposed to details of events like these?

Damon: My grandmother died when I was 20 years old. She had been diagnosed with cancer a year earlier. They tried chemotherapy, but it had already spread too much. I was there at the hospital when she died.

C: I'm sorry about the loss of your grandmother.

D: Thanks. I was close with her, so I'm glad I was able to be there with her when she passed, but it was hard to watch her go.

C: It sounds like being there was meaningful for you, and I'm glad you were able to be there with her, too. Have there been any other events in your life that were really difficult or scary?

D: No.

Based on the information gathered so far, the clinician believed they had a good assessment of Damon's trauma history because of what he put on the intake forms (i.e., "N/A") and his verbal response that the death of his grandmother was difficult for him. As a result, the clinician believed that Damon did not have a history of sexual trauma as they proceeded with the intake evaluation. The clinician continued the interview, and this next excerpt comes from an assessment of Damon's family-of-origin history.

C: Now, I'd like to ask some questions about your childhood. Who raised you?

D: Mostly my mom. She and my dad divorced when I was three years old, and I only saw my dad once or twice a year after that.

C: Do you have any siblings?

D: Yeah, my mom remarried when I was 10, and I have two half-sisters.

C: How would you describe your childhood growing up?

D: It was OK. I mean, my mom did the best she could, but she had to work a lot. I spent a lot of time at my neighbor's apartment because my mom couldn't afford a regular babysitter for me.

C: What was your time like at your neighbor's apartment?

D: Uh . . . it was OK. I didn't like being over there, but I had no choice.

C: Why was it that you didn't like being at your neighbor's?

D: Sometimes he would tell me I needed to change my clothes, even though my clothes weren't dirty. He'd have me change in front of him, and he would touch himself.

C: So, the person who was supposed to be watching out for you and keeping you safe while your mom was working actually did some things that sound like they must have been confusing or scary for you.

D: Yeah, I didn't know what was going on until later.

C: How do you think this experience impacted you?

D: I remember being mad at my mom when I was little for making me go over to his apartment. But now, I realize that she didn't know what was going on and was trying to provide for me.

C: Do you think about what happened at your neighbor's apartment very often now?

D: No. I haven't thought about that in a long time.

C: Are there any activities, places, or other things that you avoid because they remind you of your neighbor?

D: No.

C: Thank you for sharing that experience with me. It sounds like those experiences resulted in some anger towards your mom when you were younger, but it doesn't seem like it's causing any problems for you at this time. Does that seem accurate to you?

D: Yeah, I agree with that.

In the preceding exchange, the clinician did not expect Damon to disclose any unwanted sexual experiences. However, while discussing his childhood, Damon disclosed child sexual abuse. There are a few key take-home messages from this exchange. First, while, at first glance, it may be easy to assume that Damon is not presenting information in a straightforward way by not disclosing these unwanted sexual experiences earlier in the intake, the way Damon labels these experiences and how they are impacting his current functioning are the more likely reasons that he did not disclose this information earlier. In particular, he may not consider these events to be "traumatic," particularly since they are not impacting his current functioning. Clients may hold different definitions of what events they consider "traumatic," with some clients considering even minor stressors traumatic, others believing only very severe incidents can be traumatic, and many falling somewhere in between. As a result, it was important that the clinician did not attempt to confront Damon about a discrepancy in reporting during this exchange. Furthermore, Damon never used the term "sexual abuse" in describing the experience, so it is not clear if Damon identifies these experiences as such. In this exchange, the clinician did not attempt to push any particular label on the experiences and instead used Damon's own language when asking follow-up questions.

Second, when Damon first began discussing spending time with his neighbor, it seemed like there was more that he was not sharing initially. The clinician used an open-ended question (i.e., "Why was it that you didn't like being at your neighbor's?") to get more information. The clinician then used a summary statement to provide validation. This reaction was important because the clinician was likely surprised to learn of child sexual abuse but reacting with surprise could send a message to Damon that he said something he "shouldn't" have said. Instead, the clinician's responses allowed Damon to share more information about his experience.

Third, the clinician assessed for mental health problems related to this child sexual abuse. While Damon was presenting for symptoms of OCD, it was important for the clinician to assess if the patient was experiencing any symptoms related to the trauma. That said, the clinician kept the assessment brief, which is important because clients may become frustrated if their assessment becomes sidetracked by topics they do not believe are relevant to their current concerns. Therefore, in this case, the clinician appropriately balanced assessment of problems secondary to the trauma while not spending too much time on it when it became clear that this does not appear to be a primary concern for the patient right now.

Finally, while not part of the exchange, one additional consideration for this exchange involves child abuse reporting requirements. This issue is discussed in more detail in the section about adult survivors of child sexual abuse in Chapter 9, but it is important that clinicians are familiar with reporting requirements in their states. If this disclosure would require the clinician to make a report, clients should be provided with information about this limit to confidentiality prior to the start of the assessment. Then, clinicians should inform clients of the reporting requirement following the disclosure and explain what information will be shared as part of the required reporting.

EXAMPLE 2

In this second example, the clinician worked in a college counseling center and had been working with a female college student, Vicky, for several sessions. Specifically, the clinician had been providing cognitive-behavioral therapy (CBT) for social anxiety disorder. Vicky did not report any history of traumatic events at intake. The following discussion took place during Vicky's sixth treatment session.

> *Clinician:* Hi, Vicky, to start out today, I want to check in on how things have been going for you since the last session.
> *Vicky:* Ummm . . . well, I don't really know.
> *C:* OK, how about just today? How are you feeling today?
> *V:* Not good. I guess I haven't been feeling very well since I woke up Sunday.
> *C:* That's helpful for me to know. When you say you haven't been feeling very well, do you mean physically, emotionally, or both?
> *V:* Mostly emotionally.
> *C:* What types of emotions have you been feeling since you woke up on Sunday?
> *V:* Lots of things—sad, anxious, and guilty.
> *C:* What do you think led to those feelings?
> *V:* Umm . . . well . . .
> *C:* These feelings started when you woke up Sunday morning?
> *V:* Yeah.
> *C:* What was different between Saturday morning and Sunday morning for you?
> *V:* Saturday night, my friends convinced me to go to a party with them. I felt really nervous about going, so I had a lot to drink to help calm me

down. I ended up talking with this guy I know from my classes—the party was at his house.

C: So, you went to a party Saturday night? What happened at the party?

V: That guy ended up inviting me to go to his room with him. I didn't really want to, but I didn't know how to say "no," so I went. We kissed for a little while, and then I told him I should go meet up with my friends. He told me I should stay with him and said if I left, he'd think I didn't like him. He said we could watch a TV show, so I stayed. About halfway through the show, he got on top of me and started kissing me again. I asked him to slow down and watch the show, but he said he couldn't keep his hands off me. I didn't know what else to say, and he just kept going. After he took my clothes off, I told him it was getting late and that I needed to get back to my friends, but he said I couldn't leave him like that after getting him so worked up. I didn't know what to do, I just froze, and he ended up having sex with me. After, I went and found my friends, and I asked them if we could go home. They agreed, and someone drove us all back to our apartments.

C: Did you tell your friends what had happened?

V: No. I didn't want to talk about it. I just wanted to go home and go to bed.

C: So, you got home, and what happened next?

V: I took a shower and went to bed. When I woke up the next morning, I felt terrible. I didn't want to have sex with him, and I know I never should have gone up to his room. I also know I'm so stupid for not just leaving when I had so many chances.

C: Vicky, I really appreciate you walking me through what's been going on since Sunday. I know the plan for this session was to continue with in vivo exposure, but I'm wondering if we should instead spend some time talking about what happened and how you've been feeling?

In this example, the clinician was expecting to have a "regular" CBT session with their patient to address symptoms of social anxiety disorder. Instead, the plan for the session was disrupted by a disclosure of sexual assault. There are several key points regarding this interaction. First, as in the example in Chapter 6 and Example 1 in this chapter, the clinician did not label the experience for Vicky. Because Vicky may not label the event as a rape or sexual assault and may not use those terms for her experience at this time, it is important that the clinician not force those terms on her.

Another important take-away from this excerpt is the importance of reacting in a nonjudgmental way to the information presented. Some clinicians may, in effort to help the patient identify ways to increase safety in the future, jump into problem solving how to drink less and how to be more assertive in sexual interactions. While well intentioned, these discussions could imply that the clinician blames Vicky for the sexual assault. Instead, the clinician uses open-ended questions to learn more about what happened.

Many clinicians on college campuses are designated as "confidential employees" (i.e., employees who do not need to report knowledge of sexual assault to the Title IX coordinator; see Chapter 9 for additional information about Title IX reporting); therefore, when clients disclose sexual assault to a mental health provider, even one working in a college counseling center, there is typically no requirement to report the incident. However, clinicians may experience urges to encourage survivors to report the incident to the police and/or to campus authorities. These urges are likely coming from a desire to help survivors get justice for what happened. However, survivors may be hesitant to report their sexual assault to the police or campus authorities for a variety of reasons (e.g., concerns about retaliation, confidentiality, effects on social groups). As a result, it is important that clinicians be prepared to help clients weigh the pros and cons of reporting and not reporting and that clinicians be respectful of clients' decisions regarding whether to report or not.

In addition, many treatment protocols, particularly CBT protocols, involve the use of agendas for the sessions and tend to have specific skills for use in specific sessions. As a result, an important skill for clinicians using these treatments is to be able to keep the client focused on the treatment goals and treatment plan. This is often necessary because patients may try to avoid engaging in exposure activities by bringing up additional stressors or difficulties. However, in this situation, the clinician recognized that flexibility with regard to the treatment plan was needed given the disclosure of sexual assault. Specifically, if the clinician had tried to guide Vicky away from talking about the sexual assault and reminded her of the exposure activity planned for the day, Vicky may have thought the clinician did not believe her experience was significant or worth talking about. That said, the clinician also presents Vicky with an option for how to spend the session. It is important to give survivors of sexual assault agency to make decisions, and it is also important to recognize that survivors will vary in what needs they will have at various times following the sexual assault. Therefore, if clinically appropriate, it can be helpful in these cases to allow the client to choose whether to continue with the planned treatment material or to delay that material for a session. If Vicky chooses to focus on discussing the sexual assault during this session, it will be important for the clinician to consider when to resume treatment for social anxiety disorder. Factors to consider when making this decision should include the frequency of sessions, the client's level of distress related to the sexual assault, the client's level of distress related to the initial presenting concern (in Vicky's case, social anxiety disorder), and what other resources are available to provide additional support.

Finally, this case demonstrates why clinicians, regardless of whether they specialize in treatment of trauma-related disorders or not, must be prepared to receive disclosures of sexual assault at any time during treatment. Furthermore, clinicians should be familiar with local resources for survivors of sexual assault (e.g., victim services agencies) so that they can be provided should such a disclosure occur and the client is in need of resources. Clinicians who work in a college counseling center should be aware of both campus and community resources, as survivors may have a preference for the type of resource or there may be barriers for accessing some of these resources (e.g., transportation off campus).

CONCLUSION

In this chapter, we provided two examples of unanticipated disclosures of sexual assault that occurred during clinical service delivery. In the first example, the disclosure occurred during the initial evaluation, but it was not expected due to the client's responses to other questions during the evaluation. In the second example, the client experienced a sexual assault between sessions and disclosed it in the next session. Both of these examples highlight the importance of clinicians taking a nonjudgmental, validating stance to receiving disclosures, even when they are not expected.

8

Case Example 3

Exposure Therapy with a Survivor of Sexual Assault

In Chapter 5, we presented a variety of considerations for working with survivors of sexual assault in psychotherapy. In this chapter, we present a case example of a clinician preparing to conduct imaginal exposure for posttraumatic stress disorder (PTSD) secondary to a sexual assault. The primary goal of this example is to demonstrate how clinicians can help clients incorporate more details into their trauma narratives and the necessity of the clinician being comfortable hearing and using sexual terms during such treatment. This chapter is not meant to teach clinicians how to conduct imaginal exposure therapy; clinicians who wish to learn to conduct imaginal exposure for PTSD should refer to other materials, such as the manuals for Prolonged Exposure (PE; Foa et al., 2019) or Trauma Management Therapy (TMT; Beidel et al., 2018), and pursue targeted trainings in how to conduct imaginal exposure.

In this example, the clinician was beginning imaginal exposure with a male veteran, Paul, who has been diagnosed with PTSD due to a sexual assault he experienced during his military service (note: pseudonyms were used for all case examples and identifying details were changed to protect confidentiality). During the assessment, Paul used the acronym MST (i.e., military sexual trauma) to label his sexual assault. The clinician was gathering the details of the event to use for imaginal exposure in future sessions. At the beginning of the session, the clinician reviewed Paul's self-report measures and completed a brief check-in with him. The clinician then explained the rationale for exposure therapy for PTSD to Paul. At this point in the session, the clinician was ready to start gathering details about the sexual assault to prepare for exposure therapy.

> *Clinician:* Now that we've talked about what imaginal exposure will involve, I want to make sure I have a really good sense of what happened during the event. To start us off, can you walk me through what happened during your MST?
>
> *Paul:* It had been a long day in training. I went to the showers to just wash away the stress of the day. I heard the door open, and I figured someone

else was coming in to shower. The next thing I knew, I was on the ground and couldn't get up. They were holding my face down on the ground. They took turns raping me. When they were done, I got up and got back in the shower and cleaned myself up.

C: Thank you for taking me through what happened. At this point, I'd like to ask some questions to help fill in more details. For the imaginal exposure, it's really important that we include as many details as possible so that when you recall the MST for imaginal exposure, it will be as vivid of a memory as possible.

P: OK ...

C: It can certainly be hard to talk about these things, but I want to make sure that you aren't avoiding any details, because avoiding only works in the short term. Plus, if you can remember the MST in lots of detail during the exposure sessions, then when the memories come up outside of sessions, you'll be able to handle those as well.

P: I guess that makes sense.

In the preceding excerpt, the clinician allowed the patient to give an overview of the event first. This overview sets the stage for the clinician to ask follow-up questions and obtain more details. It is very common for trauma survivors to provide a brief overview that does not include a lot of detail when first describing their traumatic event. It is the clinician's job to help elicit details about crucial areas. But it is helpful to get a full overview before filling in details so the clinician knows where the patient may need to expand. Also, in this excerpt, the clinician provided an explanation for why they were going to ask for more details. It is important for clients to understand why clinicians are asking for more details both to ensure they include the details when conducting the imaginal exposure in the future and to try to protect against clients interpreting these questions as blaming them or questioning what occurred.

C: So, you were in the shower, and you heard the door open. What else did you hear?

P: I heard a few guys whispering to one another.

C: Could you make out any of what they were saying?

P: Not really, not at first.

C: OK, so this is when you were thinking that whoever had come in was coming to shower too?

P: Yeah.

C: You mentioned that you couldn't make out what was being said at first. What did you hear?

P: Once they got close, I heard one of them say, "Let's teach him a lesson."

C: What did you think at that point?

P: That's when I realized that it was probably the guys who have been messing with me around base. I thought, "Crap, what are they going to pull now?"

C: What did you think they would likely do?

P: I figured they'd take my towel or something like that.

C: So, you had the thought that they might take your towel, and what happened next?

P: I heard the shower curtain get ripped open. I went to turn around, but before I could, one of them grabbed me, and they pulled me down to the ground just outside of where the water was.

C: What thoughts did you have at that point?

P: I didn't know what to think. I just kept hoping that they wouldn't hurt me too badly.

C: What sensations did you notice in your body? What emotions did you feel?

P: My heart was racing, and I felt really scared. I wanted to fight back, but three of them were holding me down.

In this preceding excerpt, the clinician elicited more details about the initial part of the assault. In particular, the clinician gathered information about thoughts and feelings Paul experienced during this part of the trauma. The information about thoughts is especially important to gather, as this information can be helpful in addressing self-blame. For example, many survivors of sexual assault experience hindsight bias that influences their level of self-blame. By identifying their thoughts from the moment, it can help survivors view their responses as more reasonable given the information they had at that time. For example, if Paul blamed himself for not acting more quickly when the perpetrators entered the bathroom, it may be helpful for Paul to remember that in the moment, he did not know who had entered, and even when he realized who it was, he initially thought their actions would be less serious (i.e., stealing his towel). Similarly, remembering physical and emotional reactions can help survivors put some of their responses into perspective as well (e.g., survivors who experienced a freeze response during the assault may benefit from recalling their emotional responses). In the next excerpt, the clinician continued to obtain more details about the event.

C: You're being held down, and you're feeling scared, hoping they don't hurt you. Do you know how many people are there?

P: There's four—the three guys holding me down and one more.

C: OK. What happens next?

P: The fourth one started raping me.

C: What exactly did he do?

P: He stuck it inside me.

C: Did he put his penis inside you or some other object? And when you say "inside you," do you mean in your anus?

P: He . . . he put his penis in my butt.

C: What did you notice in your body when this happened?

P: There was such a sharp pain. It felt like being stabbed over and over again with every thrust.

C: What thoughts did you have at this point?

P: I just kept thinking, "Why are they doing this? Please make it stop."

C: What happened next?

P: The other three each took their turn.

C: So, they traded off holding you down and raping you?

P: Yeah.

C: What did you do while this was occurring?

P: I just kept telling myself that it would be over soon. I tried to jerk my arms away once or twice, but then they just pressed harder into the tile until it felt like my wrist was going to break.

C: Did they all penetrate your butt with their penises?

P: I think so.

C: What sensations did you notice as the others took their turn raping you?

P: The pain didn't stop. The whole time I just kept thinking how I wished they would have just beaten me up.

During this portion of the discussion, the clinician asked Paul to provide a lot more detail about the portion of the assault when sexual penetration occurred. Of note, when Paul initially described this part of the trauma, he simply stated, "They took turns raping me." This wording is important, because it allows the clinician to use the term "rape" when asking follow-up questions. If Paul had not used this term, the clinician would want to be careful to use the words that Paul had used when asking follow-up questions. Also, Paul provided some details about the incident that then allowed the clinician to be more targeted in their questions. For example, Paul had identified that he was raped by more than one person and that the perpetrators were "guys," which meant the clinician then knew there was more than one assailant, as well as the gender of the individuals who raped Paul. If Paul had been vaguer in his description, the clinician would have needed to be mindful to not make assumptions about the number of assailants or their gender. Additionally, it is very common for survivors of sexual assault to provide limited information about the sexual contact portion of the trauma. Many individuals do not feel comfortable discussing sexual contact (consensual or nonconsensual), and individuals with PTSD tend to avoid talking about their traumatic events. Thus, this combination often results in patients sharing limited details about this portion of the sexual assault. In this excerpt, the clinician modeled for the patient some of the language to use to describe the sexual penetration when they asked if the penetration was with the perpetrator's penis or an object and by confirming where Paul was penetrated. Furthermore, the clinician asked for additional details about sensations and thoughts during this portion of the traumatic event. Clinicians should also ask about additional sensory details (i.e., sights, sounds, smells, tastes, touch sensations) to help make the trauma narrative as immersive as possible. Again, due to the tendency to want to avoid thinking and talking about sexual incidents and trauma, patients often limit details to keep this portion as short as possible, and clinicians must demonstrate a willingness to hear details about this part of the assault and encourage patients to share these details.

In these discussions, it is very important that clinicians keep questions as open-ended as possible in order to allow the patient to fill in details accurately. When an open-ended question is not possible, the clinician should provide a few alternative possibilities to ensure that they are not making assumptions about what occurred. For example, when the clinician first asked Paul about the penetration, they asked if the perpetrator used his penis or an object to avoid making assumptions one way or the other. Furthermore, open-ended questions can help avoid implying blame toward the client regarding the sexual assault. As an example, asking whether the survivor fought back could led the patient to infer that the clinician believes they should have done more to protect themselves. In contrast, the clinician in this example used an open-ended question by asking what Paul did during the assault, leaving it open for him to provide a wide range of responses.

C: How did you know when they were finished?

P: I could tell when each guy was done, because I'd feel them switching off on who was holding my left arm down. When the fourth one got off me, I prayed that it was over. One of them said, "I hope that teaches you to not get us all screwed into more PT again in the future."

C: What happened then?

P: They finally all got off me, and then one of them threw a towel on top of me and told me to clean myself up. I couldn't bring myself to move. I was in so much pain. I heard their footsteps go to the door and I heard the door close behind them. I finally pulled myself back up off the floor.

C: What did you notice when you stood up?

P: I reached back, and my butt was covered in blood, and it was sticky. I slowly walked back under the water and tried to clean myself up. I then toweled off and tried to return to the barracks and walk normally so no one would notice anything off, which made my butt hurt even more.

C: So, after they left, you noticed your butt was covered in blood, and was the sticky substance semen?

P: Yeah.

C: I really appreciate you providing me all of these additional details about your MST.

P: Yeah. I've never told anyone those details before. I try to push all of that out of my head because I worry that if I start thinking about it, then it won't stop. It's hard to talk about it.

C: It's completely reasonable to not want to think about something that is so hard to talk about. But since it keeps coming back to you in unwanted thoughts and nightmares, having all these details will really help us to do the exposure as effectively as possible to try to help reduce those symptoms.

In this final section, the clinician again introduced sexual terminology (i.e., "semen") into the conversation to model use of this language for the client. The clinician also continued to mirror the language that Paul used (e.g., use of the word "hard" rather than "traumatic" to describe the incident). Also, the clinician provided validation that Paul's avoidance up until this time made sense while also integrating in why avoidance does not work in the long term, which provided an explanation for why the details are necessary.

CONCLUSION

In this chapter, we reviewed excerpts from a discussion a clinician had with a patient regarding their sexual assault to obtain more details about the experience, which will allow them to more effectively conduct imaginal exposure therapy. In general, it is important for clinicians to be willing to listen to details about unwanted sexual contact and to ask questions to get more details about what that contact involved. Furthermore, clinicians should be careful in their language and wording of questions during exposure therapy to avoid labeling experiences in a way that is not consistent with how the client conceptualizes the event and to minimize the likelihood that the client will believe the clinician blames them for the assault happening.

REFERENCES

Beidel, D. C., Frueh, B. C., Neer, S. M., & Lejuez, C. W. (2018). *Trauma Management Therapy*. Unpublished manuscript, University of Central Florida.

Foa, E. B., Hembree, E. A., Rothbaum, B. O., & Rauch, S. A. M. (2019). *Prolonged Exposure therapy for PTSD: Emotional processing of traumatic experiences: Therapist guide* (2nd ed.). Oxford University Press.

9

Special Considerations
for Various Populations

The goal of this book was to provide clinicians and other professionals with practical advice for handling client disclosures of sexual assault. While previous chapters have provided broad advice to guide work with survivors of sexual assault, in this chapter, we provide guidance on working with various specific populations. Specifically, we discuss issues clinicians need to consider when working with children and adolescents, adults who disclose child sexual abuse, male survivors of sexual assault, survivors who identify as a sexual and/or gender minority, survivors of color, and military personnel and veterans. Finally, we provide specific advice for clinicians who may have multiple roles in educational settings and for clinicians who provide group therapy to survivors of sexual assault.

CONSIDERATIONS FOR CHILD AND ADOLESCENT
SURVIVORS OF SEXUAL ABUSE AND SEXUAL ASSAULT

When assessing sexual abuse and sexual assault in children and adolescents, it is important that clinicians consider developmental level when choosing assessment measures. Specifically, clinicians must consider issues such as whether the child can complete written self-report measures; whether pictures, dolls, or other visual aids are needed; and what terminology is most appropriate for the child's developmental level. Furthermore, clinicians should consider whether to obtain information from others (e.g., parents, guardians) as part of the assessment process. Clinicians should also be mindful of not guiding children's responses or suggesting there are "correct" responses to the questions, given that children are particularly suggestible (see Saywitz & Lyon, 2002, for a review). See Chapter 4 for more information about assessment of sexual abuse and sexual assault in children and adolescents.

Additionally, clinicians working with children and adolescents must be familiar with the child abuse reporting laws and procedures in the state or states in which they practice. All states in the United States require health care professionals, including mental health practitioners, to report cases of suspected child abuse and neglect; however, these statutes have been criticized for being vague (Kalichman & Brosig, 1993). Furthermore, states vary in what experiences meet criteria for child abuse and neglect (e.g., whether exposure to domestic violence constitutes child abuse) and the definition of statutory rape (e.g., whether young adults can engage in sexual activity with adolescents within a certain age range, sometimes referred to as "Romeo and Juliet laws").

Because of the requirement to report child abuse, clinicians should ensure that this limit to confidentiality is discussed with parents or guardians during the consent process and with children and adolescents during the assent process. Clinicians should ensure they use developmentally appropriate language when discussing this limit with children and adolescents. Clinicians also need to have a plan for deciding whether they will tell the child/adolescent and parent/guardian in advance if a report will be made. In some cases, the clinician may want to inform the family in advance in an attempt to maintain trust in the relationship. However, if the clinician believes that knowing about the report in advance may put the child, clinician, or another individual in danger, the clinician likely should not tell the family in advance. Furthermore, some agencies may have additional steps and guidelines that the clinicians they employ are to follow when they need to make a report, such as notifying supervisors and completing specific documentation.

An additional point of consideration when working with children and adolescents who have experienced child sexual abuse is integrating strategies to increase safety into the treatment plan. Identifying ways to increase future safety is a key component of Trauma-Focused Cognitive Behavior Therapy (TF-CBT; Cohen et al., 2017). The purpose of this component is to reduce the likelihood of revictimization (see Walker et al., 2019, for a review). Specifically, children are encouraged to identify individuals who can help keep them safe and how those individuals can help them (Hendricks et al., n.d.). Because parents or caregivers are commonly involved in TF-CBT, this information can be shared with them to help enhance the child's physical safety and sense of safety.

CONSIDERATIONS FOR ADULT SURVIVORS OF CHILDHOOD SEXUAL ABUSE

Clinicians should be prepared for adult patients to disclose a history of child sexual abuse during an assessment of trauma history. Specifically, more than one-fourth of female adolescents and more than one out of 20 male adolescents reported experiencing at least one incident of sexual abuse or sexual assault before the age of 17 (Finkelhor et al., 2014). Furthermore, 31% of women admitted to an inpatient facility reported a history of child sexual abuse (Cloitre et al., 1996). As a result, just by the nature of these base rates, clinicians will work with survivors of child sexual abuse regardless of the treatment facility where they work or their particular specialty.

Similar to when working with child and adolescent survivors of child sexual abuse, clinicians must be familiar with whether disclosure of previous abuse by an adult patient must be reported in their state. Importantly, in some states, whether there is current risk to a child (e.g., an adult client who reported child sexual abuse perpetrated by a parent has a younger sibling living with the parent) will affect whether the abuse needs to be reported. Clinicians should consult with the state agency that receives child abuse reports, legal counsel, or counsel at their malpractice insurance company for specific guidance.

Furthermore, adult survivors of child sexual abuse tend to experience additional symptoms beyond those that are typical of survivors of sexual assault that occurs in adulthood. According to the resource loss model of childhood abuse trauma, children have limited resources to cope when traumatic events occur (Cloitre et al., 2006). For example, a child's developmental level impacts their ability to identify risk and protect themselves; additionally, their cognitive abilities may limit their ability to process the event. Furthermore, if the perpetrator was a caregiver, the child may not have the ability to escape the abusive situation. In addition to the limited resources the child may have to cope with the trauma, the child is likely to lose important resources related to psychosocial development. Specifically, children who experience childhood abuse are likely to experience loss in three areas: "(1) loss of healthy attachment, (2) loss of effective guidance in the development of emotional and social competencies, and (3) loss of support and connection to the larger social community" (Cloitre et al., 2006, p. 5). Similarly, in the theoretical rationale underlying contextual therapy for survivors of prolonged child abuse, it is noted that even when the perpetrator is not a parent or primary caregiver, many children exposed to significant child abuse are raised in family environments that do not provide adequate support for psychosocial development (see Gold, 2008, for a review).

Consistent with the idea that childhood abuse is associated with losses that impact psychosocial development, a study of women found that while both women who experienced sexual assault in adulthood and women who experienced sexual trauma in both childhood and adulthood had high rates of posttraumatic stress disorder (PTSD), women who experienced both child and adult sexual assault reported higher levels of affect regulation difficulties (e.g., dissociative symptoms, alexithymia, suicide attempts) and interpersonal problems than women who experienced sexual assault in adulthood only and women who had not experienced sexual assault (Cloitre et al., 1997). Furthermore, research has found that affective regulation difficulties and interpersonal problems are positively associated with functional impairment among survivors of child abuse, even after accounting for the effect of PTSD symptoms (Cloitre et al., 2005). As a result, adult survivors of child sexual abuse may need additional treatment strategies to address affective and interpersonal difficulties. Depending on the client's needs, clinicians may wish to consider treatments such as Skills Training in Affective and Interpersonal Regulation (STAIR; Cloitre et al., 2006) and Dialectical Behavior Therapy (Linehan, 1993), depending on the degree of difficulties the client is experiencing in these domains.

CONSIDERATIONS FOR MALE SURVIVORS

Although the sexual violence literature on victims has disproportionately focused on women, and women are indeed at higher risk of being sexually assaulted, approximately one in every 10 sexual assault victims identifies as male (Anderson et al., 2018; Artime et al., 2014; Department of Justice, 2013). Additionally, male survivors evidence lower rates of reporting and care seeking than female survivors (Weiss, 2010). Ultimately, all formal sources of support need to be prepared to effectively work with male survivors and actively work to reduce barriers to care. Much of the information presented throughout this book applies to all survivors of sexual assault regardless of gender. However, there are some unique features that arise when working with male survivors.

First, male survivors of sexual assault are more likely to be unacknowledged survivors, meaning that they more often use nonvictimizing language to describe what happened to them (e.g., "It was a miscommunication because I was drunk"; Reed et al., 2020). This trend is thought to stem from the propensity for men to more strongly believe rape myths, which may impact how they conceptualize themselves and their own victimization. Ultimately, the high rates of unacknowledged rape among male survivors likely serve as a barrier to reporting the crime and receiving needed services (Reed et al., 2020; Weiss, 2010). The advice given in Chapter 2 regarding how to work with unacknowledged survivors applies to male survivors. However, it is important for formal sources of support to know that male survivors are more likely to use nonvictimizing language when describing the incident(s) and that their conceptualization of what happened to them should not detract from the fact that they were assaulted.

Second, there are rape myths specific to male survivors that may impact interactions with professionals. For example, if during Cognitive Processing Therapy (Resick et al., 2017), a male survivor endorses the belief "men cannot be raped," the clinician should consider the role of this thought in perpetuating the client's current symptoms, and it may be appropriate to challenge that cognition. Furthermore, prior research has found that male survivors are more likely to experience self-blame for their assault (Davies, 2002), which may be due to endorsement of beliefs that men should be able to protect themselves. When this belief is present, it will need to be addressed during treatment. Although the psychotherapy techniques discussed in Chapter 5 apply to working with male survivors, it may be appropriate to also provide psychoeducation on the rates and impact of sexual assault among men to normalize the client's experience and to challenge male-specific rape myths. In a related point, formal sources of support need to be mindful of ways they may unintentionally communicate that they adhere to male rape myths. For example, if a clinician or police officer asks why the male survivor did not physically fight back against the assailant more, it may communicate that the clinician or officer believes that a man should be able to defend himself against sexual violence. Although the clinician or officer may simply be collecting information about the incident, this question may inadvertently communicate that they do not believe that the assault happened or that the survivor is to blame for what happened. As discussed in Chapter 2, professionals need to be careful about the wording they use and need to clearly communicate the purpose of questions/ statements.

Third, sexual assault is more likely to lead to confusion and concerns related to sexuality among male survivors, particularly if the incident was perpetrated by another man or men, the client identifies as heterosexual, and the survivor experienced arousal and/or orgasm (Bullock & Beckson, 2011; Davies, 2002). Therefore, providers should be prepared to discuss these concerns with clients, comfortably talk about sexual activity and sexuality, and educate the survivor on physiological reactions. Related to sexual orientation, men who identify as gay and are sexually assaulted may worry that health care providers will respond to them in a homophobic way or that police may not take their disclosure seriously (Jackson et al., 2017; National Coalition of Anti-Violence Programs, 2010). These concerns may exaggerate existing mistrust of authorities and make them less likely to report the crime or seek services. We will further discuss issues related to sexual orientation later in the chapter.

Fourth, male survivors of sexual assault are more likely to delay seeking medical and mental health care (Donne et al., 2017). In addition to common reasons that survivors in general delay seeking services, male survivors also report concerns related to feeling emasculated, worrying others will make assumptions about their sexual orientation, fearing they will be perceived as weak for needing help, and feeling embarrassed that they experienced arousal during the incident (Porta et al., 2018; Sable et al., 2006). Generally speaking, providers need to be aware that traditional gender norms related to masculinity create barriers to disclosure and access to services for male survivors. Formal sources of support should ensure that policies and procedures do not explicitly or implicitly exclude male survivors (e.g., definitions of rape that specify vaginal-penile penetration) and should participate in community engagement programs to change cultural scripts surrounding sexual assault perpetrated against men.

Finally, finding the "right fit" between client and provider is always important. For example, in Chapter 3, we highlighted the important role of establishing rapport. However, establishing trust and finding the right clinician may be even more challenging for male survivors of sexual assault (Donne et al., 2017). Male survivors often express frustration with not being able to find a mental health professional they feel comfortable talking to or having concerns about the confidentiality of their disclosures (Donne et al., 2017; Sable et al., 2006). In a related point, because most awareness and educational materials are geared toward women, male survivors also report that they are uncertain of where they can obtain help and what services are available to them (Sable et al., 2006). Formal sources of support should more intentionally target men in their advertising materials and better communicate that they are a safe and accepting resource for all survivors, regardless of gender. To do so, materials and processes should be presented in a gender-neutral way or in a way that reflects the gender identity of the particular survivor currently being helped. Doing so will ensure that all survivors feel supported and validated. For example, when working with a survivor who identifies as male, professionals should provide information that is either gender neutral or specific to male survivors. It would be inappropriate to provide this survivor with information that is geared toward a female survivor. Professionals can locate resources for male survivors online, including the 1in6 webpage (https://1in6.org) or the male-specific sections on the Rape, Abuse & Incest National Network (https://www.rainn.org/articles/sexual-assault-men-and-boys) and the National Sexual Violence Resource Center (https://www.nsvrc.org/resource-topics/men) webpages.

CONSIDERATIONS FOR SURVIVORS WHO IDENTIFY AS GENDER AND SEXUAL MINORITIES

Given that the majority of prior studies have focused on cisgender, heterosexual female survivors, survivors who identify as LGBTQ+ have largely been overlooked in the literature. This is particularly problematic because the little research that does exist suggests that individuals who identify as a sexual or gender minority are at higher risk of sexual victimization than their cisgender, heterosexual counterparts, and the psychological impact of sexual victimization may be greater on the LGBTQ+ community (Hoxmeier, 2016; Murchison et al., 2016; Rothman et al., 2011; Sigurvinsdottir & Ullman, 2016). Women who identify as bisexual or as a lesbian, in particular, experience high rates of sexual violence, with some estimates suggesting the rate could be as high as 85% (Rothman et al., 2011). Men who identify as bisexual or gay also evidence high rates of sexual violence, with prevalence rates between 40% and 47% (Black et al., 2011). Additionally, identifying as a gender minority compounds risk for sexual assault above and beyond identifying as a sexual minority (Langenderfer-Magruder et al., 2016). Prior research has also suggested that individuals who identify as a sexual or gender minority may access mental health services more often than their cisgender and heterosexual counterparts, which indicates that all providers need to be prepared to offer effective and affirming services (Cochran et al., 2003); however, little is known specifically about disclosure and treatment seeking in the aftermath of sexual assault within the LGBTQ+ community.

Although there has been little scholarship specifically dedicated to examining disclosure among sexual assault survivors who identify as LGBTQ+, there is some preliminary evidence to suggest that LGBTQ+ survivors may receive more negative reactions to their disclosures (Binion & Gray, 2020; Koon-Magnin & Schulze, 2019). Furthermore, there may be differences in the language used by survivors. Specifically, prior research has suggested that participants who identified as non-binary (Anderson et al., 2019) or as a sexual minority (e.g., bisexual, gay, lesbian, asexual; Wilson & Newins, 2019) have significantly higher rates of acknowledged rape than heterosexual, cisgender, or transgender survivors. Therefore, disclosures by individuals who identify as non-binary or a sexual minority may be more likely to include the word "rape" than other survivors. Additionally, because acknowledged rape has been linked to increased odds of seeking care and re-porting the assault (Walsh et al., 2016), it is possible that survivors who identify as a sexual minority or as non-binary may be more likely to present for services or report the crime to authorities. In contrast, a growing body of literature has documented high levels of fear about interacting with police and hesitation to re-port crimes within the transgender community, particularly among transgender women of color (Langenderfer-Magruder et al., 2016; National Coalition of Anti-Violence Programs, 2013). This fear stems from witnessing and experiencing police violence, including physical injury, harassment, threats, and intimidation (National Coalition of Anti-Violence Programs, 2013). Overall, additional re-search is needed to better understand disclosure and reporting of sexual assault among survivors who identify as LGBTQ+ given that there may be differences within this community based on intersecting marginalized identities.

Related to rape acknowledgment, there is evidence to suggest that individuals who identify as a sexual minority or as non-binary may have higher rates of ac-knowledged rape because they are less likely to adhere to rape myths (Wilson & Newins, 2019; Worthen, 2021). Subsequently, these individuals may have fewer cognitive distortions related to rape myths. However, other sociocultural factors may create issues in how survivors who identify as sexual and gender minorities view themselves and their victimization. Specifically, many individuals who iden-tify as LGBTQ+ experience internalized homophobia and/or transphobia, such as believing they deserved to be sexually assaulted because of their sexual and/ or gender identity (Davies, 2002; Gold et al., 2007). In fact, prior research has suggested that internalized homophobia is a stronger predictor of psychological outcome following sexual assault than the severity of the victimization (Gold et al., 2007). Therefore, it is recommended that mental health providers assess for the presence and impact of internalized homophobia and transphobia on LGBTQ+ sexual assault survivors and consider challenging these maladaptive thoughts via cognitive-behavioral therapy (CBT; Binion & Gray, 2020). However, it is also important to note that individuals who identify as LGBTQ+ do in fact experi-ence high rates of discrimination, microaggressions, and harassment; therefore, clinicians need to carefully balance validating clients' realistic concerns about safety and challenging cognitive distortions that are contributing to psychosocial difficulties.

Despite existing research that has suggested that individuals who identify as LGBTQ+ may seek mental health services more often, there is also robust ev-idence demonstrating that these individuals face many barriers to accessing high-quality care and community services, including stigma, discrimination, and microaggressions (Dean et al., 2000). For example, some individuals who identify as transgender have reported that they have been denied services at rape crisis centers and counseling centers because of their gender identity and/or expres-sion (Kenagy, 2005; Seelman, 2015). Additionally, individuals who identify as a sexual or gender minority report that many providers have limited knowledge about the LGBTQ+ community and believe myths about individuals who identify as LGBTQ+ (e.g., "gay men are promiscuous;" Todahl et al., 2009). Additionally, many individuals who identify as LGBTQ+ fear that their identity will become the focus of the services and/or worry that they may be outed. Overall, individuals who identify as a sexual or gender minority perceive that community services and agencies are not equipped to help them in the aftermath of sexual assault (Todahl et al., 2009). Furthermore, within the LGBTQ+ community, survivors of color, survivors with disabilities, and survivors who are perceived to be transgender are more likely to receive unequal treatment (Todahl et al., 2009). Thus, survivors who identify as LGBTQ+ cannot be treated as a monolithic group with homogenous experiences (Binion & Gray, 2020). Instead, providers are advised to consider unique aspects of each survivor that may impact their daily experiences, the conceptualization of their assault, and, ultimately, their trajectory toward recovery.

We recommend that all formal sources of support receive training related to working with individuals who identify as sexual and gender minorities, with a particular emphasis on trainings that take both an intersectional and minority stress approach. Specifically, minority stress theory (Meyer, 2003) may help providers better understand how daily discrimination and stigma compound to impact functioning. In fact, prior research has demonstrated that daily heterosexism longitudinally predicts PTSD symptoms among women who identify as a sexual minority above and beyond trauma exposure (Dworkin et al., 2018). Furthermore, an intersectional framework may help professionals better comprehend how systems of privilege and oppression intersect to impact survivors (e.g., transgender women of color; Crenshaw, 1991). Furthermore, all policies, materials, and procedures should be reviewed and revised to be as inclusive as possible. Clinicians should also closely monitor their own heteronormative and cisnormative beliefs and assumptions when interacting with survivors. In a related point, many disciplines have guidelines and recommendations for serving clients who identify as LGBTQ+, and providers should familiarize themselves with those suggestions (e.g., American Psychological Association, 2012, 2015). Providers should also understand that survivors' sexual and/or gender identities are likely only relevant in terms of how to respectfully interact with the person (e.g., use correct pronouns, phrase questions in an inclusive way). Their identity should not become a central focus point of the services unless the survivor specifically brings the topic up or the provider deems that it is clinically relevant. Finally, if appropriate, agencies and organizations should advertise and communicate that they are LGBTQ+ affirming and inclusive so that all survivors know they can safely receive services.

CONSIDERATIONS FOR BLACK, INDIGENOUS, AND PEOPLE OF COLOR (BIPOC) SURVIVORS OF SEXUAL ASSAULT

As has been mentioned previously, the sexual assault literature has overwhelmingly focused on White survivors. Furthermore, individuals who are racial and ethnic minorities are more likely to drop out of trauma studies than non-Hispanic, White participants, which has only further biased the existing literature (Boykin et al., 2016). This disparity in research has led to numerous unanswered questions, including the exact prevalence of sexual assault within BIPOC communities. However, in general, the existing literature points to particularly heightened risk for sexual assault among BIPOC women (Bryant-Davis et al., 2009).

Similar to the sociocultural factors discussed throughout the book (e.g., rape myths, internalized homophobia), additional aspects of the context in which survivors live may impact assault disclosure, crime reporting, and treatment seeking among BIPOC survivors. Although the particular historical events, group-specific rape myths, and/or cultural influences may differ between particular racial or ethnic groups, the consequences are generally the same (e.g., underreporting of the prevalence of sexual assault, lack of visibility in scholarship, hesitancy to report or disclose sexual assault, inconsistent punishment for perpetrators). For example, the impact of slavery in the United States and associated sexual victimization of Black women is still apparent, given that men who rape White women are given harsher prison sentences than men who rape Black women (Moorti, 2002). Additionally, police officers have been found to have more negative beliefs about survivors of color (e.g., describing the survivor as uncooperative, claiming the survivor would not do well as a witness in court), which ultimately may serve as perceived barriers to the investigation process and can impact the prosecution of the crime (Shaw et al., 2016). Additional barriers to disclosure among Black women include stereotypes related to sexuality, systems of oppression, lack of resources, and the perceived need to protect Black men who perpetrate sexual assault (McNair & Neville, 1996). Another example is that Latina women often do not disclose sexual assault because they fear they will not be believed due to stereotypes that characterize Latina women as flirtatious and hypersexual (Feagin & Feagin, 1996). And, in fact, White, non-Hispanic sexual assault survivors receive higher levels of empathy from disclosure recipients than Latina sexual assault survivors (Jimenez & Abreu, 2003). To truly understand the experiences of racial and ethnic minority survivors, providers need to appreciate that in addition to more universal reasons (e.g., fear of not being believed, minimizing the assault), there may be more nuanced reasons that BIPOC survivors do not report or disclose their assault. As discussed earlier in reference to internalized homophobia, it may be appropriate for clinicians to address cognitive distortions that stem from these stereotypes within the context of CBT. However, given the frequency of discrimination, violence, and harassment within BIPOC communities (e.g., excessive use of force by police), clinicians also need to delicately balance validating the client's legitimate concerns about safety and challenge cognitive distortions that impact functioning.

Best practices for working with sexual assault survivors of color emphasize the importance of accounting for the individual's context and the relevant sociocultural factors when providing services. More specifically, agencies and organizations should engage in community outreach programs to connect with BIPOC communities (Smyth et al., 2006). Given the high levels of mistrust, particularly toward police, providers could create opportunities to engage with particular communities to establish a trusting relationship. For example, police officers could meet with a church community to allow the members to meet the officers and for the police officers to provide helpful information on accessing services. Furthermore, such interactions would allow agencies and organizations to engage in educational and preventive programming with the community. Additionally, formal sources of support should engage in cultural competence training and provide culturally informed services, with an emphasis on utilizing an intersectional approach (Crenshaw, 1991; Smyth et al., 2006). Providers should be mindful of any stereotypes or preexisting beliefs related to race or ethnicity that may impact their ability to work with particular survivors. For example, providers who believe sexualized stereotypes about Black women may be more likely to blame a Black woman for her assault (West, 1995). In fact, prior research has demonstrated that Black survivors tend to be blamed more than White survivors (Donovan, 2007). Agencies and organizations should also more actively hire diverse staff members, including for leadership positions. This is important because BIPOC survivors are often hesitant to seek services at agencies and organizations with predominantly White staff members because they fear that their experiences will not be understood (Washington, 2001). Finally, providers need to understand that sexual assault survivors of color may need more comprehensive services and may be less aware of resources that are available to them (Smyth et al., 2006). Therefore, providers are encouraged to make appropriate referrals for additional services and to help survivors establish the services they may benefit from.

CONSIDERATIONS FOR MILITARY AND VETERAN POPULATIONS

Military service increases one's risk for experiencing a sexual assault (Zinzow et al, 2007). Specifically, prior research has suggested that the rate of sexual assault during deployment among women is approximately double the lifetime prevalence of sexual assault among women in the general population (Suris & Lind, 2008). Similarly, the rate of sexual assault during deployment among men is between five and nine times higher than the rate of sexual assault among men in the general population (Suris & Lind, 2008). Additionally, more recent data suggest that the documented rate of sexual assault within the military is increasing, which appears to largely be due to increased awareness of the issue and improved reporting procedures (Department of Defense, 2020). Given the high, and increasing, rate of sexual assault, providers who work with military service members and veterans need to be well versed in survivor-centered care (Department of Defense, 2020; Wilson, 2018). Furthermore, evidence has suggested that social support, including social reactions, may be a particularly powerful predictor of psychosocial difficulties for military personnel and veterans, compared to civilians (Brewin et al., 2000; Zalta et al., 2021). Providers should be mindful that transitions related to deploying or returning home will lead to changes in social support (Hinojosa

& Hinojosa, 2011; Riggs & Riggs, 2011). Consequently, these changes may impact disclosure of sexual assault. For example, someone who was sexually assaulted while deployed in a combat zone may feel uncomfortable disclosing the assault to their available support network during deployment and also may not believe they are able to discuss the incident with their support network at home. Given the many challenges military personnel and veterans face when seeking support, providers need to be prepared to have supportive and affirming conversations about sexual assault.

Although it is important to know that most veterans and military service members are satisfied with the disclosure conversations they have with professionals regarding sexual assault, there are some areas of concern (Street et al., 2019). Most notably, because anonymous surveys find higher rates of military sexual trauma than data collected through the Veterans Health Administration or military, it appears that many military service members and veterans are hesitant to disclose their sexual assaults to providers (Street et al., 2019). Research has demonstrated that, regardless of the skill of the provider or the circumstances of the interaction, many veterans are resistant to disclosing sexual assault. Hesitancy to disclose is particularly common among male veterans because of traditional gender norms (Street et al., 2019; Turchik et al., 2013). Many veterans and military service members also report typical concerns about disclosing sexual assault, such as embarrassment, fear about being believed, and perceptions the disclosure will not be helpful (Patterson et al., 2009; Street et al., 2019). The good news is that even when veterans are resistant to talking about sexual assault, they still recognize the process as important and beneficial (Street et al., 2019).

In addition to the more typical concerns related to disclosure that apply to most sexual assault survivors, military service members and veterans also report some unique fears related to the hierarchical nature of the military and the inherent power differential (Ilies et al., 2003). Due to the hierarchical structure, reports of sexual assaults in the military go to the service member's commanding officer, who has a wide range of options for how to proceed with the case (Department of Defense, 2004). Therefore, many survivors are hesitant to report their victimization out of fear of how it will be handled, concerns about potential negative impact on their career, or worry that the report will not be kept confidential (Burns et al., 2014; Dardis et al., 2018). Furthermore, many survivors report that they found their options of who to disclose to less than ideal or indicate confusion about how to report an assault (Blais et al., 2018; Dardis et al., 2018). Also unique to the military is the hypermasculine environment that perpetuates rape myths (Dardis et al., 2018; Stander & Thomsen, 2016). This culture can contribute to negative reactions toward survivors by other service members and lead to self-blame. In a related point, survivors of military sexual assault appear to be particularly at risk for high levels of self-stigma, which may involve negative beliefs about what the assault says about them as a person and/or negative attitudes about the impact of the assault on them (Andresen & Blais, 2019). And, prior research has found that self-stigma among military sexual assault survivors leads to nondisclosure out of fear of appearing weak (Andresen & Blais, 2019). Furthermore, the perpetrators of military sexual assault tend to be other service members with whom the survivor must continue to work and live, which can lead to concerns about future safety, possible retaliation, and the potential for negative social consequences. If the perpetrator is a service member from the survivor's own unit, then this can be particularly distressing because units are taught to function as a trusting, cohesive group who rely on each other for safety and security (Freyd et al., 2007). If the perpetrator is a member of the survivor's unit, the survivor is less likely to disclose the assault to others (Blais et al., 2018).

In terms of provider recommendations, prior research has again confirmed the importance of establishing a trusting relationship because veterans have been found to be more likely to disclose to a provider they trust and with whom they have an ongoing relationship (Blais et al., 2018; Street et al., 2019). Additionally, some research has suggested that veterans are more likely to disclose the assault if verbally asked about sexual victimization than when they completed a self-report questionnaire (Street et al., 2019). However, other studies have found higher reporting rates on anonymous surveys (Bovin et al., 2019). This discrepancy points to the importance of using an assessment battery and collecting information via multiple modalities and instruments. Veterans also reported that they were more satisfied with providers who used clear and concise language when discussing sexual assault, as well as those who offered definitions for the terms they used (Street et al., 2019). It may also be helpful to provide psychoeducation so that service members and veterans better understand how assessment information will be used (Bovin et al., 2019). Veterans also reported that they were happier with provider interactions if the provider displayed compassion, was nonjudgmental, and allowed the veteran to have some control over the interaction (Street et al., 2019). Veterans also appreciated when providers promptly provided information on resources and treatment options, as well as provided psychoeducation on how common assault is and the typical reactions (Bovin et al., 2019; Street et al, 2019). Providers are also encouraged to review the Veterans Health Administration recommendations for screening for military sexual trauma (Bell, 2017).

CONSIDERATIONS FOR CLINICIANS WITH MULTIPLE ROLES IN EDUCATIONAL SETTINGS

In addition to child abuse reporting requirements, individuals in educational settings may be required to comply with compelled disclosure policies. Title IX prohibits discrimination on the basis of sex in educational activities when the institution receives federal funding (Office for Civil Rights, 2015). The 2011 "Dear Colleague letter" (Ali, 2011) made it clear that sexual assault is considered a form of sexual discrimination and that institutions must act promptly to respond to reports of sexual assault. A 2014 Q&A document (Lhamon, 2014) clarified that schools are considered to have notice of sexual violence (and therefore have an obligation to respond) if a responsible employee knows of the incident, and this document also provided guidance on the definition of a responsible employee.

Given that institutions are required to act when a responsible employee knows of the incident, responsible employees must disclose knowledge of a sexual assault to the Title IX coordinator at the institution, even if the survivor does not want it disclosed to the Title IX coordinator. While Title IX applies to all educational institutions that receive federal funding, this section will focus on institutions of higher education, as the topic of compelled disclosure has been a topic of significant discussion recently and because most college students are adults, meaning many sexual assaults on college campuses are not incidents of child abuse and do not involve mandated reporting to child protection agencies.

Because of Title IX requirements, colleges and universities have developed policies regarding compelled disclosure to identify responsible employees at their institution. A study of university sexual assault policies revealed that 88% of the policies examined in the study named all or almost all university employees as responsible employees (Holland et al., 2018). Even in policies in which all or almost all university employees are identified as responsible employees, these campus policies also identify confidential employees, which commonly include licensed health care providers, including mental health providers. Confidential employees do not have to disclose sexual violence they learn about as part of their role as a confidential employee. As a result, mental health providers in higher education settings should ensure that their role or facility is noted in campus policies as being a confidential resource (Newins, 2019). For example, directors of mental health training clinics on college campuses should ensure their facility is recognized as a confidential resource if they treat college students. Furthermore, some mental health providers on college campuses may have multiple roles, some of which are confidential and some of which are not. For example, a clinician who provides services in the campus counseling center will likely be a confidential resource in that role, but if they also teach a course, they may be considered a responsible employee in their role as an instructor. As a result, these individuals should ensure they understand their reporting responsibilities under each role and identify ways to help students understand how to distinguish when they are serving in each role and how that distinction will affect compelled disclosure (Newins, 2019). Furthermore, when serving as a responsible employee, individuals who may interact with survivors of sexual assault should consider how to provide information about their duties as a responsible employee to students in order to allow students to make an informed decision about what information they wish to share. For example, instructors may consider including a statement about compelled disclosure in their syllabi and/or discussing compelled disclosure at the outset of each course. For more information about ethical considerations about compelled disclosure for psychologists in higher education settings, see Newins (2019).

CONSIDERATIONS FOR GROUP THERAPY

Survivors of sexual assault may benefit from group therapy either in place of or in addition to individual therapy. Group therapy may be beneficial for survivors of trauma, including survivors of sexual assault, because it can provide an opportunity to connect with others to reduce feelings of isolation and increase trust (Foy et al., 2001). Group therapy can also validate an individual's experiences and responses through interacting with others who have also experienced trauma. Furthermore, group treatment may be more cost effective in some settings. There are several factors that clinicians should consider when using group therapy with survivors of assault.

First, clinicians should consider whether the group will be restricted to survivors of sexual assault or if the group will include survivors of other types of trauma (or even individuals who have not experienced trauma). While some models of group therapy are specific to survivors of sexual assault (see Vandeusen & Carr, 2003), some group treatments are not specific to survivors of sexual assault (e.g., cognitive processing therapy, psychoeducation groups on trauma in general, skills training groups to address depression). As a result, clinicians should consider the content of the group material as well as the degree to which details of traumatic events will be disclosed when deciding whether survivors of sexual assault need a separate group or could be combined with other patients. Furthermore, clinicians should consider the distribution of various characteristics among group members. For example, if a survivor of sexual assault will be the only survivor of that type of trauma and the only woman in a group of male trauma survivors, the clinician should consider how these differences will impact the survivor's ability to engage in the group. Clients should also be invited to participate in the decision-making process. For example, if the client will be the only survivor of sexual assault in a skills training group that the clinician believes would be helpful for the survivor, the clinician should have a discussion with the client about the pros and cons of various options (e.g., participating in the group anyway, receiving the skills training individually, not receiving the skills training, delaying skills training until additional survivors of sexual assault can participate).

Second, clinicians need to consider whether trauma details will be discussed and to what degree in the group setting. For example, groups focused on coping and support often do not involve sharing trauma details, while other groups do involve discussing the trauma in order for clients to process the trauma and to obtain support from other survivors (Foy et al., 2001; Vandeusen & Carr, 2003). After determining whether sharing trauma details is relevant to the group content, clinicians should ensure clients are aware of expectations to share (or not share) details of their traumatic event during group sessions. Additionally, clients should be provided with a rationale for why trauma details are to be discussed (e.g., to help get perspectives and support from others about the traumatic event) or not be discussed (e.g., to avoid sharing details that could be upsetting to other clients).

Third, discussions of expectations regarding confidentiality in group therapy are particularly important when working with survivors of sexual assault because of the high levels of shame and stigma survivors face. In our experience, we have found it helpful to encourage clients to share the content of psychoeducational and skills training group sessions with their support network while asking clients to keep confidential who else is in group with them and what other group members said during group.

CONCLUSION

Although this chapter is by no means exhaustive, our goal was to offer more targeted advice and special considerations for working with particular sexual assault survivors or in particular settings. There are countless other character- istics of survivors and/or settings that may be relevant to the disclosure process, and providers should do their best to minimize barriers to services. For example, survivors who live in rural communities may face additional challenges in terms of finding a trained professional to whom they feel comfortable disclosing and may have particularly heightened concerns about confidentiality (Donne et al., 2017; Johnson & Hiller, 2019). Ultimately, the recommendations offered in this chapter can be summarized by encouraging providers to take into account the unique characteristics of the survivor, the setting, and their role in order to best serve and support the survivor.

REFERENCES

Ali, R. (2011). *Dear Colleague letter.* U.S. Department of Education, Office for Civil Rights. https://www2.ed.gov/about/offices/list/ocr/letters/colleague-201104.pdf

American Psychological Association. (2012). Guidelines for psychological practice with lesbian, gay, and bisexual clients. *American Psychologist, 67*(1), 10–42. https://doi. org/10.1037/a0024659

American Psychological Association. (2015). Guidelines for psychological practice with transgender and gender non-conforming people. *American Psychologist, 70*(9), 832–864. https://doi.org/10.1037%2Fa0039906

Anderson, R. E., Cahill, S. P., & Delahanty, D. L. (2018). The psychometric properties of the Sexual Experiences Survey–Short Form Victimization (SES-SFV) and charac- teristics of sexual victimization experiences in college men. *Psychology of Men and Masculinity, 19*(1), 25–34. https://doi.org/10.1037/men0000073

Anderson, R. E., Tarasoff, L. A., VanKim, N., & Flanders, C. (2019). Differences in rape acknowledgement and mental health outcomes across transgender, non-binary, and cisgender bisexual youth. *Journal of Interpersonal Violence.* Advance online publica- tion. https://doi.org/10.1177/0886260519829763

Andresen, F. J., & Blais, R. K., (2019). Higher self-stigma is related to lower likelihood of disclosing military sexual trauma during screening in female victims. *Psychological Trauma: Theory, Research, Practice, and Policy, 11*(4), 372–378. https://doi.org/ 10.1037/tra0000406

Artime, M. T., McCallum, E. B., & Peterson, Z. D. (2014). Men's acknowledgment of their sexual victimization experiences. *Psychology of Men and Masculinity, 15*(3), 313–323. https://doi.org/10.1037/a0033376

Bell, M. E. (2017). Military sexual trauma [Psych/Armor online course]. https://psycharmor.org/courses/military-sexual-trauma-2/

Binion, K., & Gray, M. J. (2020). Minority stress theory and internalizing homophobia among LGB sexual assault survivors: Implications for posttraumatic adjustment. *Journal of Loss and Trauma*, *25*(5), 454–471. https://doi.org/10.1080/15325024.2019.1707987

Black, M. C., Basile, K. C., Breiding, M. J., Smith, S. G., Walters, M. L., Merrick, M. T., Chen, J., & Stevens, M. R. (2011). The National Intimate Partner and Sexual Violence Survey (NISVS): 2010 summary report. https://www.cdc.gov/violenceprevention/pdf/nisvs_report2010-a.pdf

Blais, R. K., Brignone, E., Fargo, J. D., Galbreath, N. W., & Gundlapalli, A. V. (2018). Assailant identity and self-reported nondisclosure of military sexual trauma in partnered women veterans. *Psychological Trauma: Theory, Research, Practice, and Policy*, *10*(4), 470–474. https://doi.org/10.1037/tra0000320

Bovin, M. J., Black, S. K., Kleiman, S. E., Brown, M. E., Brown, L. G., Street, A. E., Rosen, R. C., Keane, T. M., & Marx, B. P. (2019). The impact of assessment modality and demographic characteristics on endorsement of military sexual trauma. *Women's Health Issues*, *29*(Suppl 1), S67–S73. https://doi.org/10.1016/j.whi.2019.03.005

Boykin, D. M., London, M. J., & Orcutt, H. K. (2016). Examining minority attrition among women in longitudinal trauma research. *Journal of Traumatic Stress*, *29*(1), 26–32. https://doi.org/10.1002/jts.22066

Brewin, C. R., Andrews, B., & Valentine, J. D. (2000). Meta-analysis of risk factors for posttraumatic stress disorder in trauma-exposed adults. *Journal of Counseling and Clinical Psychology*, *68*(5), 748–766. https://doi.org/10.1037//0022-006X.68.5.748

Bryant-Davis, T., Chung, H., & Tillman, S. (2009). From the margins to the center: Ethnic minority women and the mental health effects of sexual assault. *Trauma, Violence, & Abuse*, *10*(4), 330–357. https://doi.org/10.1177/1524838009339755

Bullock, C. M., & Beckson, M. (2011). Male victims of sexual assault: Phenomenology, psychology, physiology. *Journal of the American Academy of Psychiatry and the Law*, *39*(2), 197–205.

Burns, B., Grindlay, K., Holt, K., Manski, R., & Grossman, D. (2014). Military sexual trauma among US servicewomen during deployment: A qualitative study. *American Journal of Public Health*, *104*(2), 345–349. https://doi.org/10.2105/AJPH.2013.301576

Cloitre, M., Cohen, L. R., & Koenen, K. C. (2006). *Treating survivors of childhood abuse: Psychotherapy for the interrupted life*. Guilford Press.

Cloitre, M., Miranda, R., Stovall-McClough, K. C., & Han, H. (2005). Beyond PTSD: Emotion regulation and interpersonal problems as predictors of functional impairment in survivors of childhood abuse. *Behavior Therapy*, *36*(2), 119–124. https://doi.org/10.1016/S0005-7894(05)80060-7

Cloitre, M., Scarvalone, P., & Difede, J. (1997). Posttraumatic stress disorder, self- and interpersonal dysfunction among sexually retraumatized women. *Journal of Traumatic Stress*, *10*(3), 437–452. https://doi.org/10.1023/a:1024893305226

Cloitre, M., Tardiff, K., Marzuk, P. M., Leon, A. C., & Portera, L. (1996). Childhood abuse and subsequent sexual assault among female inpatients. *Journal of Traumatic Stress*, *9*(3), 473–482. https://doi.org/10.1007/BF02103659

Cochran, S. D., Mays, V. M., & Sullivan, J. G. (2003). Prevalence of mental disorders, psychological distress, and mental health services use among lesbian, gay, and bisexual adults in the United States. *Journal of Consulting and Clinical Psychology*, *71*(1), 53–61. https://doi.org/10.1037//0022-006x.71.1.53

Cohen, J. A., Mannarino, A. P., & Deblinger, E. (2017). *Treating trauma and traumatic grief in children and adolescents* (2nd ed.). Guilford Press.

Crenshaw, K. (1991). Mapping the margins: Intersectionality, identity politics, and violence against women of color. *Stanford Law Review*, *43*(6), 1241–1299. https://doi.org/10.2307/1229039

Dardis, C. M., Reinhardt, K. M., Foynes, M. M., Medoff, N. E., & Street, A. E. (2018). "Who are you going to tell? Who's going to believe you?" Women's experiences disclosing military sexual trauma. *Psychology of Women Quarterly*, *42*(4), 414–429. https://doi.org/10.1177/0361684318796783

Davies, M. (2002). Male sexual assault victims: A selective review of the literature and implications for support services. *Aggression and Violent Behavior*, *7*(3), 203–214. https://doi.org/10.1016/S1359-1789(00)00043-4

Dean, L., Meyer, I. H., Robinson, K., Sell, R. L., Sember, R., Silenzio, V.M. B., Bowen, D. J., Bradford, J., Rothblum, E., White, J., Dunn, P., Lawrence, A., Wolfe, D., & Xavier, J. (2000). Lesbian, gay, bisexual, and transgender health: Findings and concerns. *Journal of the Gay and Lesbian Medical Association*, *4*(3), 102–151. https://doi.org/10.1023/A:1009573800168

Department of Defense. (2004). Task force report on care for victims of sexual assault. https://archive.defense.gov/news/May2004/d20040513SATFReport.pdf

Department of Defense. (2020). Department of Defense annual report on sexual assault in the military: Fiscal year 2019. https://media.defense.gov/2020/Apr/30/2002291660/-1/-1/1/1_department_of_defense_fiscal_year_2019_annual_report_on_sexual_assault_in_the_military.PDF

Department of Justice. (2013). *Female victims of sexual violence, 1994–2010*. Office of Justice Programs, Bureau of Justice Statistics. https://www.bjs.gov/content/pub/pdf/fvsv9410.pdf

Donne, M. D., DeLuca, J., Pleskach, P., Bromson, C., Mosley, M. P., Perez, E. T., Mathews, S. G., Stephenson, R., & Frye, V. (2017). Barriers to and facilitators of help-seeking behavior among men who experience sexual violence. *American Journal of Men's Health*, *12*(2), 189–201. https://doi.org/10.1177/1557988317740665

Donovan, R. A. (2007). To blame or not to blame: Influences of target race and observer sex on rape blame attribution. *Journal of Interpersonal Violence*, *22*(6), 722–736. https://doi.org/10.1177/0886260507300754

Dworkin, E. R., Gilmore, A. K., Bedard-Gilligan, M., Lehavot, K., Guttmannova, K., & Daysen, D. (2018). Predicting PTSD severity from experiences of trauma and heterosexism in lesbian and bisexual women: A longitudinal study of cognitive mediators. *Journal of Counseling Psychology*, *65*(3), 324–333. https://doi.org/10.1037/cou0000287

Feagin, J. R., & Feagin, C. B. (1996). *Racial and ethnic relations*. Prentice Hall.

Finkelhor, D., Shattuck, A., Turner, H. A., & Hamby, S. L. (2014). The lifetime prevalence of child sexual abuse and sexual assault assessed in late adolescence. *Journal of Adolescent Health*, *55*(3), 329–333. https://doi.org/10.1016/j.jadohealth.2013.12.026

Foy, D. W., Eriksson, C. B., & Trice, G. A. (2001). Introduction to group interventions for trauma survivors. *Group Dynamics: Theory, Research, and Practice, 5*(4), 246–251. https://doi.org/10.1037//1089-2699.5.4.246

Freyd, J. J., DePrince, A. P., & Gleaves, D. H. (2007). The state of betrayal trauma theory: Reply to McNally—Conceptual issues and future directions. *Memory, 15*(3), 295–311. https://doi.org/10.1080/09658210701256514

Gold, S. D., Marx, B. P., & Lexington, J. M. (2007). Gay male sexual assault survivors: The relations among internalized homophobia, experiential avoidance, and psychological symptom severity. *Behavior, Research, and Therapy, 45*(3), 549–562. https://doi.org/10.1016/j.brat.2006.05.006

Gold, S. N. (2008). Benefits of a contextual approach to understanding and treating complex trauma. *Journal of Trauma & Dissociation, 9*(2), 269–292. https://doi.org/10.1080/15299730802048819

Hendricks, A., Cohen, J. A., Mannarino, A. P., & Deblinger, E. (n.d.) *Your very own TF-CBT workbook*. https://tfcbt.org/wp-content/uploads/2014/07/Your-Very-Own-TF-CBT-Workbook-Final.pdf

Hinojosa, R., & Hinojosa, M. S. (2011). Using military friendships to optimize post-deployment reintegration for male Operation Iraqi Freedom/Operation Enduring Freedom veterans. *Journal of Rehabilitation Research and Development, 48*(10), 1145–1148. https://doi.org/10.1682/JRRD.2010.08.0151

Holland, K. J., Cortina, L. M., & Freyd, J. J. (2018). Compelled disclosure of college sexual assault. *American Psychologist, 73*(3), 256–268. https://doi.org/10.1037/amp0000186

Hoxmeier, J. C. (2016). Sexual assault and relationship abuse victimization of transgender undergraduate students in a national sample. *Violence and Gender, 3*(4), 202–207. https://doi.org/10.1089/vio.2016.0008

Ilies, R., Hauserman, N., Schwochau, S., & Stibal, J. (2003). Reported incidence rates of work-related sexual harassment in the United States: Using meta-analysis to explain reported rate disparities. *Personnel Psychology, 56*(3), 607–631. https://doi.org/10.1111/j.-1744-6570.2003.tb00752.x

Jackson, M. A., Valentine, S. E., Woodward, E. N., & Pantalone, D. W. (2017). Secondary victimization of sexual minority men following disclosure of sexual assault: "Victimizing me all over again." *Sexuality Research and Social Policy, 14*(3), 275–288. https://doi.org/10.1007/s13178-016-0249-6

Jimenez, J., & Abreu, J. (2003). Race and sex effects on attitudinal perceptions of acquaintance rape. *Journal of Counseling Psychology, 50*(2), 252–256. https://doi.org/10.1037/0022-0167.50.2.252

Johnson, I. D., & Hiller, M. L. (2019). Rural location and relative location: Adding community and context to the study of sexual assault survivors' time until presentation for medical care. *Journal of Interpersonal Violence, 34*(14), 2897–2919. https://doi.org/10.1177/0886260516663900

Kalichman, S. C., & Brosig, C. L. (1993). Practicing psychologists' interpretations of and compliance with child abuse reporting laws. *Law and Human Behavior, 17*(1), 83–93. https://doi.org/10.1007/BF01044538

Kenagy, G. P. (2005). The health and social service needs of transgender people in Philadelphia. *International Journal of Transgenderism, 8*(2–3), 49–56. https://doi.org/10.1300/J485v08n02_05

Koon-Magnin, S., & Schulze, C. (2019). Providing and receiving sexual assault disclosures: Findings from a sexually diverse sample of young adults. *Journal of Interpersonal Violence, 34*(2), 416–441. https://doi.org/10.1177/0886260516641280

Langenderfer-Magruder, L., Walls, N. E., Kattari, S. K., Whitfield, D. L., & Ramos, D. (2016). Sexual victimization and subsequent police reporting by gender identity among lesbian, gay, bisexual, transgender, and queer adults. *Violence and Victims, 31*(2), 320–331. https://doi.org/10.1891/0886-6708.VV-D-14-00082

Lhamon, C. (2014, April 29). Questions and answers on Title IX and sexual violence. U.S. Department of Education. https://www2.ed.gov/about/offices/list/ocr/docs/qa-201404-title-ix.pdf

Linehan, M. M. (1993). *Cognitive-behavioral treatment of borderline personality disorder.* Guilford Press.

McNair, L., & Neville, H. (1996). African-American women survivors of sexual assault: The intersection of race and class. *Women & Therapy, 18*(3), 107–118. https://doi.org/10.1300/J015v18n03_10

Meyer, I. H. (2003). Prejudice, social stress, and mental health in lesbian, gay, and bisexual populations: Conceptual issues and research evidence. *Psychological Bulletin, 129*(5), 674–697. https://doi.org/10.1037/0033-2909.129.5.674

Moorti, S. (2002). *Color of rape: Gender and race in television's public spheres.* State University of New York Press.

Murchison, G. R., Boyd, M. A., & Pachankis, J. E. (2016). Minority stress and the risk of unwanted sexual experiences in LGBQ undergraduates. *Sex Roles, 77*(3–4), 221–238. https://doi.org/10.1007/s11199-016-0710-2

National Coalition of Anti-Violence Programs. (2010). Hate violence against the LGBTQ communities in the U.S. in 2009. https://avp.org/wp-content/uploads/2017/04/2011_NCAVP_HV_Reports.pdf

National Coalition of Anti-Violence Programs. (2013). Lesbian, gay, bisexual, transgender, queer, and HIV-affected: Intimate partner violence in 2012. https://avp.org/wp-content/uploads/2017/04/ncavp_2012_ipvreport.final_.pdf

Newins, A. R. (2019). Ethical considerations of compelled disclosure of sexual assault among college students: Comment on Holland, Cortina, and Freyd (2018). *American Psychologist, 74*(2), 248–249. https://doi.org/10.1037/amp0000363

Office for Civil Rights. (2015). *Title IX and sex discrimination.* U.S. Department of Education. https://www2.ed.gov/about/offices/list/ocr/docs/tix_dis.html

Patterson, D., Greeson, M., & Campbell, R. (2009). Understanding rape survivors' decisions not to seek help from formal social systems. *Health & Social Work, 34*(2), 127–136. https://doi.org/10.1093/hsw/34.2.127

Porta, C. M., Johnson, E., & Finn, C. (2018). Male help-seeking after sexual assault: A series of case studies informing sexual assault nurse examiner practice. *Journal of Forensic Nursing, 14*(2), 106–111. https://doi.org/10.1097/JFN.0000000000000204

Reed, R. A., Pamlanye, J. T., Truex, H. R., Murphy-Neilson, M. C., Kunaniec, K. P., Newins, A. R., & Wilson, L. C. (2020). Higher rates of unacknowledged rape among men: The role of rape myth acceptance. *Psychology of Men & Masculinities, 21*(1), 162–167. https://doi.org/10.1037/men0000230

Resick, P. A., Monson, C. M., & Chard, K. M. (2017). *Cognitive processing therapy for PTSD: A comprehensive manual.* Guilford Press.

Riggs, S. A., & Riggs, D. S. (2011). Risk and resilience in military families experiencing deployment: The role of the family attachment network. *Journal of Family Psychology*, *25*(5), 675–687. https://doi.org/10.1037/a0025286

Rothman, E. F., Exner, D., & Baughman, A. L. (2011). The prevalence of sexual assault against people who identify as gay, lesbian, or bisexual in the United States: A systematic review. *Trauma, Violence, & Abuse*, *12*(2), 55–66. https://doi.org/10.1177/1524838010390707

Sable, M. R., Danis, F., Mauzy, D. L., & Gallagher, S. K. (2006). Barriers to reporting sexual assault for women and women: Perspectives of college students. *Journal of American College Health*, *55*(3), 157–162. https://doi.org/10.3200/JACH.55.3.157-162.

Saywitz, K. J., & Lyon, T. D. (2002). Coming to grips with children's suggestibility. In M. L. Eisen, J. A. Quas, & G. S. Goodman (Eds.), *Personality and clinical psychology series. Memory and suggestibility in the forensic interview* (pp. 85–113). Lawrence Erlbaum Associates Publishers.

Seelman, L. L. (2015). Unequal treatment of transgender individuals in domestic violence and rape crisis programs. *Journal of Social Service Research*, *41*, 307–325. https://doi.org/10.1080/01488376.2014.987943

Shaw, J., Campbell, R., & Cain, D. (2016). The view from inside the system: How police explain their response to sexual assault. *American Journal of Community Psychology*, *58*(3–4), 446–462. https://doi.org/10.1002/ajcp.12096

Sigurvinsdottir, R., & Ullman, S. E. (2016). Sexual orientation, race, and trauma as predictors of sexual assault recovery. *Journal of Family Violence*, *31*(7), 913–921. https://doi.org/10.1007/s10896-015-9793-8

Smyth, K., Goodman, L., & Glenn, C. (2006). The full-frame approach: A new response to marginalized women left behind by specialized services. *American Journal of Orthopsychiatry*, *76*(4), 489–502. https://doi.org/10.1037/0002-9432.76.4.489.

Stander, V. A., & Thomsen, C. J. (2016). Sexual harassment and assault in the U.S. military: A review of policy and research trends. *Military Medicine*, *181*(1 Suppl), 20–27. https://doi.org/10.7205/MILMEDD-15-00336

Street, A. E., Shin, M. H., Marchany, K. E., McCaughey, V. K., Bell, M. E., & Hamilton, A. B. (2019). Veterans' perspectives on military sexual trauma-related communication with VHA providers. *Psychological Services*. Advance online publication. https://doi.org/10.1037/ser0000395

Suris, A., & Lind, L. (2008). Military sexual trauma: A review of prevalence and associated health consequences in veterans. *Trauma, Violence, & Abuse*, *9*(4), 250–269. https://doi.org/10.1177/1524838008324419

Todahl, J. L., Linville, D., Bustin, A., Wheeler, J., & Gau, J. (2009). Sexual assault support services and community systems: Understanding critical issues and needs in the LGBTQ community. *Violence Against Women*, *15*(8), 952–976. https://doi.org/10.1177/1077801209335494.

Turchik, J. A., McLean, C., Rafie, S., Hoyt, T., Rosen, C. S., & Kimerling, R. (2013). Perceived barriers to care and provider gender preferences among veteran men who have experienced military sexual trauma: A qualitative analysis. *Psychological Services*, *10*(2), 213–222. https://doi.org/10.1037/a0029959

Vandeusen, K. M., & Carr, J. L. (2003). Recovery from sexual assault: An innovative two-stage group therapy model. *International Journal of Group Psychotherapy*, *53*(2), 201–223. https://doi.org/10.1521/ijgp.53.2.201.42815

Walker, H. E., Freud, J. S., Ellis, R. A., Fraine, S. M., & Wilson, L. C. (2019). The prevalence of sexual revictimization: A meta-analytic review. *Trauma, Violence, & Abuse*, *20*(1), 67–80. https://doi.org/10.1177/1524838017692364

Walsh, K., Zinzow, H. M., Badour, C. L., Ruggiero, K. J., Kilpatrick, D. G., & Resnick, H. S. (2016). Understanding disparities in service seeking following forcible versus drug- or alcohol-facilitated/incapacitated rape. *Journal of Interpersonal Violence*, *31*(14), 2475–2491. https://doi.org/10.1177/0886260515576968

Washington, P. A. (2001). Disclosure patterns of Black female sexual assault survivors. *Violence Against Women*, *7*(11), 1254–1283. https://doi.org/10.1177/10778010122183856

Weiss, K. G. (2010). Male sexual victimization: Examining men's experiences of rape and sexual assault. *Men and Masculinities*, *12*(3), 275–298. https://doi.org/10.1177/1097184X08322632

West, C. M. (1995). Mammy, Sapphire, and Jezebel: Historical images of Black women and their implications for psychotherapy. *Psychotherapy: Theory, Research, Practice, and Training*, *32*(3), 458–466. https://doi.org/10.1037/0033-3204.32.3.458

Wilson, L. C. (2018). The prevalence of military sexual trauma: A meta-analysis. *Trauma, Violence, & Abuse*, *19*(5), 584–597. https://doi.org/10.1177/1524838016683459

Wilson, L. C., & Newins, A. R. (2019). Rape acknowledgment and sexual minority identity: The indirect effect of rape myth acceptance. *Psychology of Sexual Orientation and Gender Diversity*, *6*(1), 113–119. https://doi.org/10.1037/sgd0000304

Worthen, M. G. F. (2021). Rape myth acceptance among lesbian, gay, bisexual, and mostly heterosexual college students. *Journal of Interpersonal Violence*, *36*(1–2), NP232–NP262. https://doi.org/10.1177/0886260517733282

Zalta, A. K., Tirone, V., Orlowska, D., Blais, R. K., Lofgreen, A., Klassen, B., Held, P., Stevens, N. R., Adkins, E., & Dent, A. L. (2021). Examining moderators of the relationship between social support and self-reported PTSD symptoms: A meta-analysis. *Psychological Bulletin*, *147*(1), 33–54. http://dx.doi.org/10.1037/bul0000316

Zinzow, H. M., Grubaugh, A. L., Monnier, J., Suffoletta-Maierle, S., & Frueh, B. C. (2007). Trauma among female veterans: A critical review. *Trauma, Violence, & Abuse*, *8*(4), 384–400. https://doi.org/10.1177/1524838007307295

10

Final Thoughts on Best Practices

Sexual assault is a unique crime. Survivors face the difficult task of not only having to convince others that a crime was committed but also demonstrating that they are not to blame for what happened to them (Aherns, 2006; Burt, 1980; Pollard, 1992; Ward, 1995). Consequently, in addition to the psychosocial consequences of the assault (e.g., posttraumatic stress disorder, depression), survivors are also impacted by the sociocultural context in which they and their disclosure recipients live (e.g., rape myths, toxic masculinity, homophobia, transphobia, racial and/or ethnic discrimination). As was discussed throughout this book, it is important to use a contextual model to consider all of the factors that influence how survivors conceptualize what happened to them, whether or not they disclose the incident to others, and how others respond to their disclosures. Professionals need to also understand how these factors may serve as barriers to survivors seeking and receiving high-quality and affirming services. In the prior chapters, we presented specific advice for particular providers (e.g., mental health professionals, police officers), job-related duties (e.g., assessment, psychotherapy), settings (e.g., colleges, military), and survivor populations (e.g., male survivors; child survivors). Here, we would like to offer some final thoughts on more general recommendations for professionals who work with sexual assault survivors.

First, all formal support providers should engage in ongoing training geared toward educating themselves about the psychological impact of trauma and best practices for discipline-specific activities and policies. The ways in which professionals respond to and interact with survivors, as well as their policies (e.g., definition of sexual assault) and practices (e.g., sexual assault nurse examiner [SANE] exam), have a powerful influence on survivors' post-assault recovery (Campbell et al., 1999). It is possible that some formal support providers are unaware of the ways in which they may be inadvertently harming survivors and potentially leading to secondary victimization. This inadvertent harm may occur because many of society's problematic attitudes and beliefs about sexual assault are so engrained that providers may not even be cognizant that they themselves adhere to these myths. Receiving training may reduce the likelihood that formal sources of support contribute to post-assault difficulties. One recommendation would be to reach out to local victim advocacy organizations or rape crisis centers to inquire about whether they offer such trainings or have recommendations for other agencies who provide trainings. It would also be good for providers to establish a relationship with the staff at victim advocacy organizations to learn about the services they provide and to be prepared to refer survivors to these community resources in the future. Ultimately, it is the responsibility of providers to ensure they are adequately trained to effectively support survivors while executing their job-related duties.

Second, the disciplines that serve sexual assault survivors need to make intersectionality theory and minority stress theory central tenets in their work. Increasingly, there is evidence that sociocultural factors, such as sexism, homophobia, transphobia, and racism, markedly impact the disclosure process and ultimately influence survivor recovery. We firmly believe that having an understanding of how intersecting identities affect an individual's experience within systems of oppression and power will contribute to higher-quality care for sexual assault survivors, as well as lead to more diversity among providers (Buchanan & Wiklund, 2020). We recommend that providers acknowledge that they are cultural beings who hold sociocultural beliefs; as a result, they should engage in self-reflection on how these beliefs may impact how they interact with sexual assault survivors and deliver services (American Psychological Association, 2017). Training programs need to better incorporate intersectionality, social justice, and issues related to diversity in the education that they provide to trainees, and continuing education opportunities need to be made available to employees (American Psychological Association, 2017). Providers are encouraged to seek consultation from knowledgeable colleagues, and supervisors should model how to provide affirming and inclusive care (American Psychological Association, 2017). Ultimately, incorporating intersectionality and social justice into our training and service delivery will create a more welcoming environment for prospective trainees, current trainees, providers, and sexual assault survivors. Buchanan and Wiklund (2020) stated that "[c]linical psychological science must change or die" (p. 324) as they articulated that the field must better integrate intersectionality and social justice in order to stay relevant. We argue that this needed shift extends beyond clinical psychology to include all fields that work with sexual assault survivors (and even beyond that).

Third, there needs to be greater societal awareness of the scope and impact of sexual assault. Media campaigns (e.g., MeToo movement), community events (e.g., Take Back the Night), and school programming (e.g., sex education) have the potential to reach wide audiences and shift the public narrative on sexual assault. In particular, these messages and programs need to focus on reducing rape myths, expanding definitions of sexual violence, and challenging traditional gender norms. This goal is particularly important because adherence to rape myths has been linked to how survivors conceptualize their victimization, how much disclosure recipients blame victims, and, ultimately, whether survivors report the crime and seek help (Aherns et al., 2007; Grubb & Turner, 2012; Reed et al., 2020; Wilson & Newins, 2019). The advantage to intervening in society in such a multifaceted way is that victim blaming would be reduced in both informal and formal sources of support, which would broaden the available network of helpers for survivors.

Fourth, providers are encouraged to display and offer emotional support to survivors while completing their discipline-specific tasks (e.g., a police officer conducting an interview with a survivor, a medical professional completing testing for sexually transmitted infections with a survivor, a mental health professional conducting an assessment of psychological symptoms with a survivor). Although there may be individual differences in how survivors perceive some reactions from disclosure recipients (e.g., telling the survivor to "move on"), there is consensus among sexual assault survivors that validation and emotional support are perceived as positive and helpful (Campbell et al., 2001; Dworkin et al., 2018). Furthermore, validating the survivor and conveying genuine empathy may in fact offset the impact of the stressful and/or unpleasant service elements that may otherwise be associated with secondary victimization (Stenius & Veysey, 2005). For example, conveying validation and empathy during a SANE exam many minimize the distress experienced by a survivor. As noted earlier, the manner in which services are delivered is often more impactful in predicting survivor outcomes than the services themselves.

Fifth, screening and assessing for sexual assault should be considered a best practice within the mental and physical health fields (see Chapter 4 for recommendations regarding assessing sexual assault history). This recommendation is based on prior research that has suggested that most survivors only disclose sexual assault after they are directly asked about it (Aherns et al., 2007). If providers fail to ask about sexual assault, then they may be missing an important factor that is contributing to the client's level of functioning. However, it is also important to keep in mind that some survivors feel more comfortable disclosing victimization experiences on self-report surveys rather than verbally during an interview and vice versa. Therefore, providers should rely on an assessment battery that asks about trauma exposure through multiple avenues and be sure to carefully follow up on any discrepancies in reporting. Simply put, providers who are unaware of the client's trauma history cannot provide relevant services or referrals. In a related point, providers who believe they are ill prepared to effectively work with any particular sexual assault survivor should be prepared to make an appropriate referral and help the survivor quickly access those services.

Sixth, formal sources of support need to be aware that survivors may be struggling to cope with the psychosocial consequences of both the trauma and the events related to the trauma (Campbell et al., 1999). For example, receiving a negative reaction from another disclosure recipient may lead to self-blame and exacerbate the survivor's distress. A survivor who perceived a previous mental health clinician as cold and insensitive may be less likely to seek future services. Ultimately, professionals need to be mindful of not only the impact of the trauma on survivors, but also how their post-assault experiences may be contributing to their current difficulties. Specific to the mental health field, mental health professionals should not focus on the traumatic incident to the exclusion of other potentially contributing factors, and they may need to adjust their therapeutic approach to address all of the relevant sources of distress.

Lastly, providers need to promote survivors' agency in advocating for themselves and empowering them to voice their needs (Worell & Remer, 1992). Professionals, even those who provide regularly scheduled services (e.g., therapist delivering weekly psychotherapy), only interact with survivors for a small amount of time. Therefore, it is vital that any interaction between formal sources of support and sexual assault survivors validate the survivor, educate the survivor on the impact of trauma, identify and challenge any adherence to rape myths, and identify and reinforce any effective coping strategies displayed by the survivor (Worell & Remer, 1992).

For most survivors, recovery following sexual assault is a lifelong process that will ebb and flow in response to other stressors, reminders of the trauma, social reactions, and sociocultural factors. Working with sexual assault survivors can be both rewarding, when you see the positive impact of your services on survivors, and challenging, when you consider the uphill battle for survivors created by the contexts in which we exist. As scholars, we are encouraged by the gains that have been made within the disciplines that serve sexual assault survivors, as well as within society as a whole. However, we also recognize that we have more work to do.

REFERENCES

Aherns, C. E. (2006). Being silenced: The impact of negative social reactions on the disclosure of rape. *American Journal of Community Psychology*, 38(3-4), 263–274. https://doi.org/10.1007/s10464-006-9069-9

Aherns, C. E., Campbell, R., Ternier-Thames, N. K., Wasco, S. M., & Sefl, T. (2007). Deciding whom to tell: Expectations and outcomes of rape survivors' first disclosures. *Psychology of Women Quarterly*, 31(1), 38–49. https://doi.org/10.1111/j.1471-6402.2007.00329.x

American Psychological Association. (2017). *Multicultural guidelines: An ecological approach to context, identity, and intersectionality.* http://www.apa.org/about/policy/multicultural-guidelines.pdf

Buchanan, N. T., & Wiklund, L. O. (2020). Why clinical science must change or die: Integrating intersectionality and social justice. *Women & Therapy*, 43(3-4), 309–329. https://doi.org/10.1080/02703149.2020.1729470

Burt, M. (1980). Cultural myths and supports for rape. *Journal of Personality and Social Psychology*, 38(2), 217–230. https://doi.org/10.1037//0022-3514.38.2.217

Campbell, R., Ahrens, C. E., Sefl, T., Wasco, S. M., & Barnes, H. E. (2001). Social reactions to rape victims: Healing and hurtful effects on psychological and physical health outcomes. *Violence and Victims*, 16(3), 287–302. https://doi.org/10.1891/0886-6708.16.3.287

Campbell, R., Sefl, T., Barnes, H. E., Aherns, C. E., Wasco, S. M., & Zaragoza-Diesfeld, Y. (1999). Community services for rape survivors: Enhancing psychological well-bring or increasing trauma? *Journal of Community and Clinical Psychology, 67*(6), 847–858. https://doi.org/10.1037//0022-006x.67.6.847

Dworkin, E. R., Newton, E., & Allen, N. E. (2018). Seeing roses in the thorn bush: Sexual assault survivors' perceptions of social reactions. *Psychology of Violence, 8*(1), 100–109. https://doi.org/10.1037/vio0000082

Grubb, A., & Turner, E. (2012). Attribution of blame in rape cases: A review of the impact of rape myth acceptance, gender role conformity and substance use on victim blaming. *Aggression and Violent Behavior, 17*(5), 443–452. https://doi.org/10.1016/j.avb.2012.06.002

Pollard, P. (1992). Judgements about victims and attackers in depicted rapes: A review. *British Journal of Social Psychology, 31*(4), 307–326. https://doi.org/10.1111/j.2044-8309.1992.tb00975.x

Reed, R. A., Pamlanye, J. T., Truex, H. R., Murphy-Neilson, M. C., Kunaniec, K. P., Newins, A. R., & Wilson, L. C. (2020). Higher rates of unacknowledged rape among men: The role of rape myth acceptance. *Psychology of Men & Masculinities, 21*(1), 162–167. https://doi.org/10.1037/men0000230

Stenius, V. M. K., & Veysey, B. M. (2005). "It's the little things": Women, trauma, and strategies for healing. *Journal of Interpersonal Violence, 20*(10), 1155–1174. https://doi.org/10.1177/0886260505278533

Ward, C. (1995). *Attitudes toward rape: Feminist and social psychological perspectives.* Sage.

Wilson, L. C., & Newins, A. R. (2019). Rape acknowledgment and sexual minority identity: The indirect effect of rape myth acceptance. *Psychology of Sexual Orientation and Gender Diversity, 6*(1), 113–119. https://doi.org/10.1037/sgd0000304

Worell, J., & Remer, P. (1992). *Feminist perspective in therapy: An empowerment model for women.* John Wiley & Sons.

For the benefit of digital users, indexed terms that span two pages (e.g., 52–53) may, on occasion, appear on only one of those pages.

Boxes are indicated by *b* following the page number.